SOME OF THE QUESTIONS
YOUR DOCTOR MAY ASK

- Did the memory problems come on slowly, over a period of years, or more quickly?
- Have physical problems, such as speech or walking difficulties, developed as well?
- What is the general health of the patient?
- Does the patient eat a balanced diet?
- Have there been changes in sleep patterns?
- Has interest in previously enjoyed activities fallen off?

Learn the most important information on diagnosing and dealing with ALZHEIMER'S

IS IT ALZHEIMER'S?

WHAT TO DO
WHEN LOVED ONES
CAN'T REMEMBER
WHAT
THEY
SHOULD

ROGER GRANET, M.D., & EILEEN FALLON

AVON BOOKS 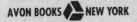 NEW YORK

The ideas, procedures, and suggestions in this book are intended to supplement, not replace, the medical advice of a trained medical professional. All matters regarding your health require medical supervision. Consult your physician before adopting the suggestions in this book, as well as about any condition that may require diagnosis or medical attention. The authors and publisher disclaim any liability arising directly or indirectly from the use of this book.

AVON BOOKS, INC.
1350 Avenue of the Americas
New York, New York 10019

Copyright © 1998 by Eileen Fallon and Roger Granet, M.D.
Published by arrangement with the authors
Visit our website at http://www.AvonBooks.com
Library of Congress Catalog Card Number: 97-94770
ISBN: 0-380-78636-2

First Avon Books Printing: July 1998

AVON TRADEMARK REG. U.S. PAT. OFF. AND IN OTHER COUNTRIES, MARCA REGISTRADA, HECHO EN U.S.A.

Printed in the U.S.A.

WCD   10 9 8 7 6 5 4 3

ACKNOWLEDGMENTS

We would like to thank our agent, Judith Riven, whose encouragement from the very conception of the project was a major factor in its being realized; our editor, Carrie Feron at Avon Books, who saw what this book could mean to those with loved ones with Alzheimer's, and Cecilia Oh, an assistant editor at Avon Books with unflagging energy; Lesley Meisoll and Laurie Martin in Dr. Granet's office for their always cheerful assistance; and the staff of the Benjamin B. Green-Field National Alzheimer's Library in the headquarters of the Alzheimer's Association in Chicago; and the Information Services Department (the "I Team") of the Cornell University Medical College Library for their invaluable reference work.

Finally, we would like to thank the following doctors for their insightful contributions, all of whom work daily to increase our knowledge in the medical areas discussed in this book and to help those confronted with memory disorders: Marvin Schwalb, Ph.D., Director of the Center for Human and Molecular Genetics at the New Jersey Medical School; Norman Relkin, M.D.,

Ph.D., Department of Neurology and Neuroscience at New York Hospital/Cornell University Medical College; and Mark Diamond, M.D., Attending Neurologist at Morristown Memorial Hospital, who has earned that most sought-after accolade, the respect and admiration of his peers.

CONTENTS

INTRODUCTION

Is It Always Alzheimer's?

The man is seventy-two. He's been forgetting things, things he should know. The worst was the other week. In his own neighborhood, *he was lost, driving around in circles until he finally found his house. And he was always sharp; now he finds himself keeping quiet in social gatherings because he can't always follow what's been said. His wife doesn't seem to notice, but one of their grown children does on a visit from out of town. She calls the local hospital and gets the name of a neurologist.*

The woman is sixty-one. She's been forgetting things, things she should know. The worst was the other week. In her own neighborhood, *she was lost, driving around in circles until she finally found her house. She's scared. Too scared to tell her husband; he wouldn't be able to cope. And her children are busy launching lives of their own. She puts off going to the doctor, making light of her concern—after all, it's probably just part of getting older, and she hates to be a bother. She'll make an appointment sometime later.*

What is the problem of our seventy-two-year-old? Because he lives in an area where there's a great deal of Lyme disease, his doctor suspects that that may be the cause of his memory difficulties. He is given, however, the full battery of tests used to diagnose memory loss, which include testing for Lyme disease if the patient lives in an area where it's known to be, or has traveled to such an area within the past few years. All the tests, including that for Lyme, come back negative, results that indicate the presence of Alzheimer's, a disease diagnosed by excluding all possible other causes of the memory problems. Yet his doctor knows that tests for Lyme often come back as false negatives, so he has the man tested again. The doctor's hunch pays off. This time the man tests positive for Lyme, and is given a heavy course of antibiotics. His mental sharpness returns.

And what about our sixty-one-year-old? Unfortunately, fear prevents her getting a diagnosis right now. The fear is that she has Alzheimer's. In reality, however, she is suffering from *vascular dementia,* a loss of memory and other mental skills often caused by *infarcts* (small strokes) or by other conditions that affect blood flow to or within the brain. After Alzheimer's, vascular dementia is the single most common cause of dementia. Diagnosis would enable doctors to treat the cause of the strokes, notably hypertension (high blood pressure). Such treatment could possibly prevent further infarcts, and thereby slow the progress of the disease. Diagnosis would also alert her grown sons and daughters to their inherited risk; they do not realize that they could significantly lower their chance of developing vascular dementia by starting an eating and exercise plan designed to prevent high blood pressure, high cholesterol levels, and obesity, the three major risk factors for both strokes and heart disease. Undiagnosed and therefore untreated,

this woman's condition will progress to the point that
she must go into a nursing home, possibly much earlier
than necessary.

The two preceding stories are true. So is the following:

*The woman is sixty-seven. She's been forgetting
things, things she should know. The worst was the
other week.* In her own neighborhood, *she was
lost, driving around in circles until she finally
found her house. She is scared. Scared but canny.
She hides her problems, and her family, experiencing the psychological phenomenon known as
denial, plays along; for instance, her grown son
takes over the household accounts, claiming that
he's working on them "with" her. They could go
on this way for years, her gradually losing more
and more of herself, and their being unable to see
it—and to prepare for the changes it must eventually cause in all their lives. But then an out-
sider's reaction breaks through the family's
denial. The woman's husband suffers a severe
stroke. In the hospital, as she maintains a vigil
with her family, she meets a young nurse. The
nurse immediately notices that something is
wrong, and refers the family to a geriatric nurse,
who in turns directs them to a memory disorder
center for diagnosis.*

And the sixty-seven-year-old? Though the testing at
the memory disorder center indicates Alzheimer's, she
is much "luckier" than the woman with vascular dementia. The center refers her to a protocol for tacrine,
later sold as Cognex, the first drug on the market developed specifically for Alzheimer's. Fortunately, she

responds extremely well to it. Later in the course of her illness she will be prescribed an antidepressant, which also works well. The social worker affiliated with the center alerts the family to the community services available to them, so she starts going to a local adult day center. As she declines somewhat and cannot be left alone in the morning to wait for the center's van, which arrives after the others in the household must leave for work, the county provides a homemaker who prepares her for her day, and stays with her until the van arrives. A proper diagnosis has led to medications and social services that delay her having to go into a nursing home for more than two years.

And those aren't the only benefits that come from diagnosis. It enables the family to plan financially for their mother's future, a vital aspect of family well-being. Finally, her grown children read about the disease, noting advances that could well help them as they age. For instance, her daughters learn of studies that link estrogen loss to Alzheimer's, and they know that, for this reason alone, they must seriously consider estrogen replacement therapy. They become tied into the Alzheimer's support and information network, and know that they will be alerted to, and will be able to take advantage of, other preventive strategies.

In short, diagnosis helps both the patient and the patient's family in a number of ways.

Not only are the three preceding stories true, the third one is that of the coauthor of this book. After her mother was diagnosed, her friends expressed their sympathy. A surprisingly large number, however, expressed fears of their own, with some variation of the following: "My mother (or father, or uncle) just isn't herself, and I know something must be wrong. But it isn't always Alzheimer's, is it? And how can we find out if it is?"

These questions made her realize the widespread need for solid, up-to-date information about Alzheimer's and other causes of severe memory problems, topics plagued by misinformation.

YOU'VE BEEN WORRIED ABOUT SOMEONE

Just like the people whose questions inspired this book, you, too, are concerned about someone. Perhaps it's your father, your mother, or even your spouse. You've noticed that he or she isn't quite the same as before, and you've started to worry. You have a number of questions, but you just don't know where to turn to have them answered.

In picking up this book, you've come to the right place. First you will read about:

- Symptoms of Alzheimer's and the disease itself.
- Other causes of dementia that show similar symptoms.
- How to find the right doctor, whether you live near or far from the patient.
- How to cope with a patient who refuses to go to the doctor.
- How the diagnosis is made.

And, after the diagnosis has been made, you'll read about:

- Treating Alzheimer's, a two-tiered approach that involves treating both the disease itself and treating the behavioral aspects of the disease, such as anxiety, depression, and agitation.
- The two currently approved drugs developed specifically for the disease.

- Drugs developed for other diseases that may be useful in treating Alzheimer's.
- Drugs developed for other diseases which treat the behavioral symptoms of Alzheimer's.
- Coping with nonmedical issues such as day care, home safety, and making the Alzheimer's patient feel safe and confident with specially designed activities.
- What a diagnosis of probable Alzheimer's means for you and your family.

Importantly, you will see that you and other caregivers also have to be taken care of, that you can successfully allocate responsibilities and cope with daily demands, and that life can be improved by some professional counseling or therapy for yourself and other family members.

You will see that you're not alone, and that a number of very valuable organizations exist specifically to provide information and the support that helps family members cope. Finally, you'll read about what the future holds, from the value of greater public awareness to the promise offered by research—including genetic research—for more effective treatments and, possibly, a cure.

In the following section you will find brief answers to the questions you have at this time, answers expanded on in the chapters that follow.

THE MOST COMMON QUESTIONS ABOUT MEMORY LOSS AND AGING

Isn't memory loss a natural part of aging?

Slight memory problems affect most people as they grow older. More and more they find themselves with an answer "on the tip of their tongues," only to discover that they can't on command bring the information forward, as it were, out of storage. All too often the answer comes a few hours or days later, when the conversation that called for it is long over. Or they will be in the middle of a sentence, only to discover that their train of thought has derailed. Or they find themselves forgetting little things—where they placed the car keys, where they left their glasses. This is called *age-related cognitive decline*, also referred to as *age-associated memory impairment*.

The basic nature of a memory disorder such as Alzheimer's is different from this sort of simple forgetting. While this kind of forgetting is an initial symptom of Alzheimer's, memory and other mental functions continue to deteriorate. You don't just forget someone's name, you forget that he or she has been part of your life for decades. You don't make normal errors in balancing your checkbook, or in a game of skill such as chess; you're starting to forget, literally, how to do these things, and the mistakes you make are of a more serious, and basic, nature. Your problems get in the way of your daily functioning. This type of progressive breaking down of mental functions is called *dementia*.

At one time, dementia was seen as a natural part of aging and viewed as a disease only in those under sixty-five. Dr. Alzheimer himself based his groundbreaking article about the disease later named for him on findings in the brain of a woman who had died in her mid-fifties. The disease incorrectly came to be referred to as *pre-senile dementia*, meaning "dementia that ocurrs before old age." The term *senile dementia* referred to dementia in those over sixty-five, and was used as recently as the 1980s.

What is Alzheimer's?

Alzheimer's is a progressive degenerative disease of the brain named for Alois Alzheimer, the physician who first wrote about it in the early years of this century. A *progressive degenerative* disease is one that becomes worse over time, and involves decay in the structure, and therefore the function, of tissue. While scientists do not yet fully understand the role of a protein called *beta amyloid* in the Alzheimer's disease process, its accumulation in the brain is always a feature of the disease. Autopsies reveal the hallmarks of Alzheimer's in the brain: *amyloid* or *neuritic plaques* (masses of beta amyloid protein outside of neurons) and *neurofibrillary tangles* (masses within neurons of altered *tau,* also a protein). It is not yet known how and why these plaques and tangles form, but it is believed that the gradual buildup of beta amyloid causes inflammation in brain tissue which, when combined with the general toxicity of beta amyloid, injures and eventually kills neurons (basic nerve cells) in the brain. The death of these neurons leads to the symptoms of Alzheimer's. You'll read more about Alzheimer's itself in Chapter Two.

What are the symptoms of Alzheimer's?

The deterioration in the functioning of the brain causes a progressive dementia, with symptoms worsening over time. When people are first affected, they show difficulties with short-term memory, forgetting, for example, the names of people they've just met, or recent conversations; basically, things they've just learned. As the disease progresses, memory problems worsen. Physicians look particularly for difficulties in at least one of the following areas, difficulties that show a decline from a previous level of functioning and that impede the person's ability to function in daily life:

- Problems with language, such as choosing the right words.
- A lessening of motor skills, such as the motions required to brush one's hair or teeth, or to button clothes.
- An inability to recognize or identify common objects at first, then even people known for years.
- Losing the ability to plan and organize, to do things in the proper sequence, to think abstractly (an ability required to learn new things, for instance).

Physicians also look for changes in personality. Does the person at times become agitated, hostile, and/or combative, and experience mood swings?

Again, they are looking for a *decline* from an earlier level of ability, and *change* itself. For instance, decades-old eating habits and sleep patterns might alter, or people might entirely lose interest in activities that used to engage them. You'll find symptoms discussed in greater depth in Chapter One.

Is it always Alzheimer's?

In a word, no.

Alzheimer's is the single most common cause of dementia, accounting for 70 to 80 percent of cases. However, a number of diseases, conditions, and substances can have dementia as a symptom. Remember the examples that opened this introduction? The dementia of the seventy-two-year-old man was actually caused by Lyme disease, and the first woman discussed had vascular dementia. Among other causes are long-term use of medications, including those frequently taken by the elderly; depression; certain metabolic problems; infections such as HIV. You'll read more about the various causes of dementia in Chapter Three.

How do we find the right doctor?

Diagnosing memory disorders is a complicated, time-consuming process, which you'll read about in Chapter Six. While a primary care physician may do part of an evaluation, it should be completed by a specialist such as a neurologist (a doctor who specializes in the care of the nervous system, which includes the brain), a geriatrician (a doctor who specializes in the care of the elderly), or a psychiatrist (a doctor who specializes in the care of emotions and behavior). And while individual physicians do diagnose memory disorders, there are also centers throughout the country that specialize in diagnosing them. The very best way to find a good doctor or center is by referral: by speaking with people who have recently dealt with the same problem you're facing, and with medical and social service professionals. You'll read about ways to contact sources that can be of help in Chapter Four. Keep in mind as well that today, with so many people in managed care health plans, you often must go through your primary care physician to reach a specialist. If you do not feel satisfied with that physician's way of dealing with this problem for any reason, you have options. You will also find them discussed in Chapter Four.

What can you do when someone with a problem refuses to see a doctor?

Due to the nature of memory disorders, many people who are suffering from them are not aware that they need help, and are often adamant about not seeing a doctor. There are ways of coping with this problem. One way is to get together several family members and say that everyone is going together to have checkups, so the one with the memory disorder does not feel stigmatized. If a family is facing tremendous resistance, another approach is to confront the person and insist that a visit to the doctor is necessary. If none of these approaches works, and you're at the end of your rope with worry that the person has become a danger to him- or herself and possibly to others (the person may set the house on fire, have a bad car accident, etc.), you may well have to turn to a last-resort option, having the person committed. Nowadays this is not a ''snake pit'' scenario but a well-regulated legal process designed to help those who are endangering themselves. You'll read about getting people to go to the doctor in Chapter Five.

How is Alzheimer's diagnosed?

There is no one, simple diagnostic test for Alzheimer's, although researchers are trying to develop one. The diagnosis of Alzheimer's is conclusive; after a full evaluation eliminates all other possible causes of a patient's symptoms, it is concluded that the probable cause is Alzheimer's. Right now the disease can only be diagnosed for certain after death through the examination of brain tissue.

The diagnostic process is a complicated, time-consuming one when Alzheimer's is suspected. A vital part of the evaluation is a complete patient history, both one prepared by the family of the dementia patient prior to the first office visit, and the one taken by the doctor during that first appointment. The patient history offers valuable clues to an experienced physician, and in the case of dementia can at times determine the order of some of the diagnostic tests. Other parts of the process are the physical examination, including vision and hearing exams; a number of medical tests, including a blood evaluation; radiologic tests such as a CT scan or MRI;

neuropsychological testing; a functional assessment (an investigation of what a person can and cannot do—get dressed, prepare a meal, etc.); and a psychosocial evaluation, which will help the family determine what caregiving steps are to be taken next. The diagnostic process is discussed in detail in Chapter Six.

Can Alzheimer's be treated?

Yes, yes, yes. In fact, two drugs developed specifically to treat Alzheimer's have already been approved by the FDA. They are Cognex (tacrine) and Aricept (donepezil). Both work by inhibiting the breakdown of the neurotransmitter acetylcholine in the brain, allowing it more time to pass on its message. (*Neurotransmitters* are chemicals that send nerve signals; *acetylcholine* is a neurotransmitter necessary for adequate memory.) *Cholinergic neurons,* the majority of those that die in the Alzheimer's disease process, are the ones that produce this neurotransmitter. Their loss reduces the amount of this vital chemical in the brain. Aricept, developed after Cognex, does not inflame the liver, as Cognex does in certain patients, and is easier to take, not requiring as many doses daily as Cognex. Both drugs temporarily improve the patient's daily functioning and mood (how much depends on the patient), and slow the progression of the disease (again, results depend on how the individual patient responds to the drug).

Other drugs, including some developed for diseases ranging from Parkinsonism to hypertension, can also be of help in treating Alzheimer's. Further, the patient's (and the patient's family's) quality of life can be improved by medications used to treat anxiety, depression, and agitation. Initial studies show that treatments such as estrogen replacement therapy and nutritional therapies can also be effective. You'll read about all these treatments in Chapter Seven.

How do we cope on a day-to-day basis?

Alzheimer's is a disease that affects those around the patient tremendously. But you can learn to deal with the problems it presents to the greatest extent possible, and help is available. First of all, a number of useful organizations are just a phone call away; some specialize in Alzheimer's, while others offer help to all those coping with a chronic illness in a loved one. Many communities provide services you will find valuable. There are also many sources to help you deal with such Alzheimer's issues as wandering, home safety, and even keeping the patient occupied and as engaged in life as possible. Finally, caregivers themselves must be cared for. You'll read about these issues, and ways to deal with them, in Chapter Eight.

Is there a cure in sight?

When you consider how much has been learned about Alzheimer's in just the past few years, you see that there is a strong foundation for breakthroughs in the years ahead; even a cure is not inconceivable, though our best hope lies, at the moment, in treating the disease. (Remember, for instance, that insulin treats but does not cure diabetes; that is merely one example of a disease that can be much better managed now than in the past.) For instance, the new *designer drugs* (medications developed to intervene in specific steps in the biochemical process of a given disease) will likely play a significant role in treatment in the very near future.

Also, due to the aging of the U.S. population, and to greater advocacy on the part of health consumers, those affected by Alzheimer's are in a stronger position now to push for necessary changes in social services. There is already evidence of such changes; for instance, the number of adult day care centers has increased tremendously in just the past few years in response to the growing need. And famous sufferers have increased public awareness.

Finally, the more we learn about Alzheimer's, the easier it will be to develop drugs to block steps in the disease process. Genetic research may one day result in a cure, but its greatest promise now is identifying these steps, knowledge that should lead to more effective treatments. You'll read about this in Chapter Nine.

THE AUTHORS' EXPERIENCE WITH DEMENTIA

Roger Granet, M.D., sees a wide range of patients in urban and suburban settings. He knows that dementia is more treatable now than ever before, that some dementias can be partly or totally reversible, and that today's medications can at minimum make those with dementia more comfortable, in itself a comfort to their families. Dr. Granet stresses however that the right treatment comes only after diagnosis.

Eileen Fallon had to learn about coping with dementia after her mother was diagnosed with Alzheimer's. Her family's experience, described in the Introduction, was that new medication, social services, and family cooperation gave them almost three treasured extra years with their mother at home, years made possible by diagnosis.

ONE

THE SYMPTOMS OF ALZHEIMER'S

MEMORY LOSS—THE EARLIEST SYMPTOM OF ALZHEIMER'S

When memory loss in older people is discussed, it's important to differentiate between the sort of mild forgetting that normally takes place as people age, referred to by doctors as age-related cognitive decline, from the more severe, progressive memory loss that is a hallmark of Alzheimer's.

With age-related cognitive decline, people find themselves misplacing things—car keys, eyeglasses, the book they are in the middle of reading—more than they would have in the past. They can also find themselves *temporarily* searching for information—a movie star's name, for instance, or the title of a play they've recently seen. These answers come to them later, usually well after the conversation that inspired them is over. These situations are more annoying than alarming, and happen to just about everyone.

Alzheimer's may, indeed, begin with this kind of forgetting, but over time, the memory problems become

1

more severe. People don't have the name of that play they saw last week on the tip of their tongues, for instance; they don't remember having seen it at all. Memory difficulties, instead of being merely annoying, become alarming.

Further, while mild forgetting is annoying to the people experiencing it, the memory problems of those who may have Alzheimer's become annoying to the people who live with them. When they start to have real difficulty with *short-term memory* (memory of events that have very recently taken place), they will ask the same question over and over again, forgetting that they've just asked it and been told the answer. For instance, the question "What day is it?" may be asked several times in just one morning. (Ways of coping with these problems of orientation are discussed in Chapter Eight.)

SYMPTOMS IN ADDITION TO MEMORY LOSS

In the Appendix, you will see the diagnostic chart doctors use to help reach a diagnosis of probable Alzheimer's. This chart is based on research into the illness, as well as clinical data (observations made by doctors when dealing with patients). Research and clinical data suggest to physicians that, in addition to a memory loss that impairs a person's ability to perform daily tasks, Alzheimer's also involves difficulties in at least one of the following four areas, difficulties that show a decline from a previous level of ability and that impede the person's functioning in everyday life:

1. Deterioration in the use of language, a condition called *aphasia* by doctors. Someone may have dif-

ficulty in pronouncing certain sounds, for instance, or may speak in a convoluted fashion, never getting to the point, or may repeatedly use unspecific words such as "thing" or meaningless sounds such as "um."

2. Deterioration in motor skills, a condition called *apraxia* by doctors. Motor skills are those required in movement. A person may, for example, lose the ability to perform certain motions, such as pouring milk into coffee, tying shoes, or waving good-bye. Skills such as writing and drawing will be affected, as will tasks such as cooking, gardening, sewing, dressing—anything requiring coordination. Motor skills are, of course, involved in walking, and the way people walk may be affected; they may start to take tiny steps, for instance, or shuffle their feet. Such a change is referred to by doctors as a *gait disturbance*.

3. Deterioration in the ability to recognize familiar objects and people, a condition called *agnosia* by doctors. People may be asked to pass the salt, for instance, and not be able to pick the salt shaker out from among other familiar objects on the table. They will also cease to recognize people known for years, even grown sons and daughters.

4. Deterioration in the ability to plan, organize, and carry out tasks requiring a number of steps, an ability referred to as *executive function* by doctors. For instance, people may no longer be able to choose clothes that make up an outfit, nor to put those clothes on in the right order, or no longer be able to prepare a meal. Their ability to learn new things is affected. While they may still be able to use the washing machine they've had for ten years, for ex-

ample, they will not be able to learn how to use a new one.

Changes in Behavior and Personality

In addition to decline in memory and in the four areas discussed in the preceding section, Alzheimer's also causes changes in behavior and personality.

Becoming anxious or depressed, or hostile, agitated, and/or possibly combative—these are some of the symptoms of Alzheimer's. Interestingly—and this is a trait much more difficult to notice than hostility—in the early stages of the disease, the opposite of hostility may be shown by someone. A basically nice, well-mannered person may become even more so, waiting on grown children hand and foot on their trips to the family home, for instance, or being very quiet but seemingly engaged when in company, smiling and nodding frequently.

Mood swings occur as well, and are frequently tied to the time of day. People are often at their most alert in the morning, then in late afternoon experience *sundowning,* an increased irritability that can grow into hostility and combativeness as the day draws to a close. (Sundowning is caused by the fatigue people with Alzheimer's feel by the late afternoon, combined with a lack of stimuli indicating that the day is, indeed, drawing to a close. Stimuli in the form of external cues could, indeed, decrease or even prevent sundowning. Among such external cues would be a large clock to enable people to confirm the late hour, as well as their hearing traditional end-of-day news and weather updates, being spoken to about dinner, and even seeing the preparation of that meal under way. Such techniques are part of *orientation therapy.*)

Also, a decrease in inhibition may be a sign of the disease. People who once had the best of manners may practically curse a blue streak in public, and state—very loudly, to the chagrin of those with them—thoughts that most of us think but don't speak aloud. "What an ugly baby!" is one such remark, for example. People may also touch themselves inappropriately in public, or make unwanted advances. In short, they lose the ability to restrain themselves, to control their impulses.

Changes in Longtime Habits and Interests

Areas in which a number of changes can take place are the daily habits of eating and sleeping. The timing of eating may change, with someone going from three meals a day to seemingly constant snacking. Tastes may change, with someone no longer eating a favorite food, and starting to devour things previously ignored. Many of those who work with Alzheimer's patients remark upon their craving for sweets, which is especially notable in those who earlier were not big sweet eaters. Sleep patterns also change; many people go to bed much earlier than in the past, but find themselves awakening hours earlier than they did before.

Lifelong interests also can wane, with hobbies and activities once eagerly engaged in falling by the wayside. These include specific activities such as gardening, card games, social dancing, and chess, for instance, as well as things perhaps not seen as activities in the same way—grocery shopping, for instance, speaking with others at a party, or engaging in long phone conversations with friends or relatives who live far away.

Interests and habits can be reflected in subtle ways, sometimes picked up on only years later by relatives of those with Alzheimer's as they look back and realize that there were some early signs of the disease that they simply didn't know enough to spot at the time. One woman recalled that her mother, who had always loved beautiful, classically understated, and expensive clothing in fine fabrics, started to dress in much cheaper fabrics and in colors she simply would not have worn for most of her life; further, her clothes just didn't "go together" as they had in the past. Another remembered going home for the holidays to find her father, a great Christmas traditionalist who had always insisted on real Christmas trees, proudly displaying his new, artificial one. And a man remembered one trip to the family home in which he'd had to bring a lot of paperwork from the office to catch up on. As he was doing so in the family study, his mother interrupted constantly, making sure he always had coffee, and asking if he needed anything else. She had always been appropriately solicitous before, he recalled, but this behavior, though pleasant, was definitely overkill.

NOTING EARLY SYMPTOMS OF ALZHEIMER'S IN LOVED ONES

In Chapter Six you'll find out how you and other family members should prepare a patient history to take to your first doctor's appointment. In the following section you'll find ways to help you determine whether someone you know has the early symptoms of Alzheimer's.

Keep in mind that what's referred to here is not the type of occasional memory lapse most people become more and more prone to as the years go by. What you're being asked to note are increasingly frequent alterations in someone's approach to everyday things, alterations that will eventually lead to impairment in day-to-day functioning. In considering the following information, consider two feelings mentioned early in this chapter—annoyance and alarm. Take particular note if you find yourself becoming annoyed by someone's lapses. There's a good chance that he or she is starting to become alarmed about what these changes mean, and could withdraw somewhat, and begin to withhold feelings of alarm from you.

Further, remember that all too often people don't really pay attention to those they've known for years, and can have difficulty even being aware of the changes wrought by Alzheimer's, which manifest in a very slow, gradual way. This is why, in fact, it is so often a grown child on a trip to the family home who notices a change in a parent, or even someone from outside the family who does not know the members that well, and whose perception isn't clouded by emotion. You may have to look at someone you're concerned about in a new, more attentive way. Compassion combined with attention to detail will be called upon here.

Memory. First and foremost, changes in this area are to be noted. Again, slight memory lapses are not a cause for alarm, but more severe, and more frequently occuring, memory problems are. In its early stages, Alzheimer's causes a great loss in recent or new information, while old memories may stay intact. For instance, a woman may not remember where her grandchild goes to grammar school, but very clearly recall where she herself went. Or a man may not merely forget where he last placed his set of keys, but forget which is the key to the house and which the car key. And people's constantly forgetting what day of the week it is, then forgetting that someone's just told them, is a frequently noted event in Alzheimer's. These memory problems are serious, and could well be the first noticeable sign that something is wrong and requires a doctor's attention.

Language. Are people speaking differently from the way they spoke in the past, at times having trouble getting a word or sound out, or perhaps speaking in long, circular sentences that never end? Do they repeat what they've just heard, instead of coming up with a sentence on their own? Do they sometimes call objects by the wrong word? Do they interchange the names of their children much more so than they may have in the past? *Listen* anew to people you've known for years, and see what changes you can note in the way they speak and use language in general.

Performing once familiar motions. What's referred to here is by no means solely a lessening of skills in very complicated motions, such as playing difficult piano pieces, accomplishing fine embroidery, or delicate painting. Alzheimer's affects a person's ability to execute simple actions of daily living—those called for, say, in personal grooming, such as brushing hair or buttoning clothes.

Recognizing familiar objects and people. An older woman may see her grown son and daughter together, and ask them how they know each other; she literally does not recognize them as her offspring. Or you may ask your father to hand you the scissors on the desk in front of him, but he merely looks right at them, not being able to pick the object out as scissors.

Planning, organizing and carrying out tasks. Has someone who used to be able to "keep herself busy" running a household started to seem at loose ends during the day, and just doesn't seem to get things done? Or perhaps the patriarch who once stage-directed the annual everybody-has-to-be-there cookout can't seem to get things going—he hasn't made up or sent out the invitations yet, hasn't yet planned his menu and ordered supplies, things he would already have done in past years. Or a person may have difficulties carrying out much simpler tasks, such as making a sandwich or making up a bed.

Eating. What you're looking for here, as elsewhere, are *changes* from years-long behavior. Someone who ate on a fairly regular schedule—breakfast at seven, lunch at noon, dinner at six-thirty, now eats seemingly haphazardly; it's almost as if he or she doesn't remember recently consuming a meal, and has become disconnected from feelings of fullness or hunger, as well as from external cues regarding meals—time of day, who is at home, presence of people in the kitchen or dining room. The choice of foods may change. For instance, someone who loved fruits and vegetables may now avoid them. And, as noted earlier, professionals with a wide experience of Alzheimer's will sometimes report that patients consume much more sugar than they did before; it seems to be an attempt to address a metabolic need, perhaps to energize the brain. However, caregivers will too often give in to the patient's desire for sweets, only to find themselves dealing with a much more agitated person once the effects of a sugar binge kick in.

Interests. Everyone has certain interests. At times they're social pursuits: dancing, parties, going out to the theater or to the movies. At others times they're more solitary: gardening, watching a favorite soap opera at the same time each weekday, reading, writing, playing an instrument—even the game of solitaire itself. Some of our activities combine social interests with more quiet ones: bridge games, for instance, or gardening club meetings. With Alzheimer's, a person's relation to these longtime interests changes. Does a man no longer go out for his weekly chess match at the local senior center? Has another man given up tending his once beloved garden? Does a woman no longer engage in those long phone conversations with her grown children?

Sleep patterns. Unfortunately, many people develop changes in sleep patterns as they age. So these changes are often a normal part of aging. They can, however, indicate Alzheimer's. Look for changes from past patterns. Does a woman now retire for the evening much earlier than before? Or is she waking much earlier, and now wandering through the house (or worse, the neighborhood) in the wee hours?

Appearance. Has someone started to dress inappropriately, be it for the season or for a particular event? Does he or she mix items of clothing that simply "don't go"? Does a woman who once meticulously applied makeup now not bother? Are appointments for haircuts further and further apart? Has personal hygiene slipped?

Temperament. Has someone who was frequently slightly difficult become much more so? Has a formerly trusting person started to show symptoms of paranoia? Has a once talkative, outgoing person become more subdued? Alternatively, has a once reserved type taken to starting up conversations with total strangers at the mall, or on line at the supermarket? Or—and this is a particularly subtle change, hard to note since it doesn't bother us as hostility does—has someone who was basically nice and accommodating become even more so?

NOTING SYMPTOMS IN A LOVED ONE— NOT AS EASY AS IT MIGHT SEEM

As previously discussed, early symptoms of Alzheimer's can be very individual and hard to recognize. Yet even as symptoms become more pronounced, those closest to the person affected often continue to be blind to them, and therefore unable to act upon them. This seeming lack of awareness is part of the psychological process called *denial*.

Denial is an *unconscious* defense mechanism used to resolve emotional conflict and relieve anxiety by disavowing thoughts, feelings, or external reality factors that are consciously intolerable. It is important to remember that people are not aware on a conscious level that they are denying the existence of facts that are fairly obvious to those with a lesser, or without any, emotional involvement in a particular situation. Denial demonstrates the power that the mind can exert over physical reality when it perceives the stakes as being high enough—and when Alzheimer's is suspected, the stakes are very high indeed.

What's at stake to the unconscious mind is, first and foremost, for a loved one to be all right. It is only human to harbor this desire, as well as to want life to go on as it always has. This emotional reality can be stronger than circumstances themselves, and can blind family members to a loved one's true state.

Yet also at stake are the advantages of diagnosis, of really taking care of the affected loved one. The sooner someone is diagnosed, the sooner medical help can start, and the sooner the family can begin to cope with the social and psychological implications of a chronic disease that will come to affect the patient's and the family's life tremendously. Further, as discussed in Chapter Three, diagnosis is vital because it may reveal that a condition other than Alzheimer's is causing the symptoms. Only after it is diagnosed can that condition be addressed.

In trying to figure out if someone is, indeed, showing symptoms and needs a doctor's attention, it helps to see how others came to acknowledge changes in a loved one. The following three anecdotes highlight different ways in which families realized that a loved one's problems were serious and required a doctor's attention. The first presents an intervention by a grown child on a visit to her parents' home. The second shows what happens when a spouse first repeatedly ignores or explains away the sorts of symptoms discussed above, then, after a diagnosis of probable Alzheimer's, tries to cope almost entirely on her own. Things eventually reach such a state that someone from outside the family or social circle must intervene, in this case, a police officer. The third, a case of the very rare early-onset Alzheimer's, features a woman whose doctor does not treat her concerns seriously, and who must then seek a new physician who will.

CAROL'S STORY: A GROWN CHILD NOTICES SYMPTOMS

Carol, seventy-one, lived on the East Coast with Tom, her husband of fifty-two years. Though she hadn't worked outside the home after marrying, she'd been a clerk in an insurance company beforehand, in a department where her aptitude for numbers served her well. In her late sixties she'd started to experience a slow decline in mental ability. It was not easy for her to remember recent events, though she could still recall her premarriage days in the insurance company with extreme clarity, remembering exactly which floor she'd worked on and her fun times with her young co-workers. In addition to this difficulty with memories of recent events and conversations, she began to act in a way that was out of character, frequently, for example, misplacing things such as important mail.

Her grown daughter, Ann, who made it home once a year from California, first became concerned about her mother via the telephone. For one thing, her father complained to her about the misplaced mail, which struck Ann as very odd, since it had always been Carol who'd kept track of things for Tom and Ann. Further, in their weekly phone conversations, Carol sounded confused at times. More and more, when Ann phoned, her father, not her mother, picked up the phone, which was also a change from the past. And when Ann once called specifically to speak with Tom on a Tuesday, her mother's evening out for bridge with friends, she was surprised to discover that Carol had not gone out, breaking a habit of seventeen years. It turned out that she had stopped going to the gatherings months before.

Concerned, Ann decided to visit her parents sooner than her next scheduled trip. Carol's appearance when Ann arrived further alerted her to the fact that something was wrong. Always a neat dresser in the past, Carol wore a mismatched floral blouse and skirt. And the blouse wasn't even buttoned right! Ann then learned that Carol was no longer keeping the family checkbook, something she'd done all along. Ann was also taken aback by her father's appearance and behavior. Generally easygoing in the past, a fifties sitcom husband and father, he looked worn out, frazzled, and he was short-tempered at times. He was obviously under stress. Tom, it seems, had started "covering" for his wife.

Covering for a loved one, Ann came to learn, happens frequently in a family when a member is in the early stages of Alzheimer's. It can be a result, at times, of a conscious wish. For example, a grown son may note that his mother's memory seems off, but he ascribes the difficulty to her being tired, or perhaps, with age, just not as sharp as she used to be; he will then step in and handle a task that seems to be daunting her. The son is aware of the problem, but hopes it will go away. Covering can also be a natural outgrowth of the process of denial. When the family has not yet consciously acknowledged that they are facing a serious problem, one or more of the members will step in and take over tasks that the affected person used to perform. The household continues to run, even if not as smoothly as before, and the illusion that all is well is preserved.

The one covering will often tell "white lies" to explain his behavior. When he took over the household finances, for instance, Tom told Carol that he really wanted to handle them because he was getting bored in retirement and wanted some work to do. Further, claiming that he'd retired partly to spend more time with her, he began to accompany her to the grocery store. And saying that he needed exercise and fresh air after years of being cooped up in an office, he took over the tending of the once-loved garden she now showed little interest in.

Fortunately, due to her friend Sean's recent experience with an uncle's Alzheimer's, Ann was aware that these symptoms could mean that her mother might well have the disease. She also knew that Sean's uncle greatly benefited from the prescription drug Aricept, the second drug developed specifically to treat Alzheimer's, and Sean had told her that the doctor said that it was best to start the drug as soon as possible in the course of the disease. Further, the uncle not only enjoyed going to an adult day center near his home, but seemed better mentally on the days he went as opposed to weekend days, when he got less stimulation. Finally, Sean's mother, who'd been taking care of her brother, benefited as well from his improved condition and from the respite the center allowed her. If, indeed, a diagnosis of probable Alzheimer's was reached, Ann wanted the same things for her mother and father—and as soon as possible.

She made an appointment with her mother's doctor. Before they went, Ann wrote down the changes she'd noted, and included a possibly relevant piece of family medical history—that Carol's paternal grandmother had been what was simply termed "senile" near the end of her life. Carol's father had died at fifty-nine, so Ann did not know if he would have developed the symptoms of dementia, but she knew that the information about Carol's grandmother would be of interest to the doctor.

After taking a patient history from Ann and Carol and then conducting some basic tests, the doctor referred Carol and Ann to a nearby memory disorder center. At the completion of the diagnostic process, they were informed that Carol had a diagnosis of probable Alzheimer's. Ann extended her stay with her parents to lay the groundwork for their getting the care and services that would ensure their future well-being, services that included enrollment at a day center recommended by people whom Ann met through the local chapter of the Alzheimer's Association, as well as proper legal advice about finances from an attorney specializing in elder law issues; the attorney was also referred by people met through the Alzheimer's Association.

*

PHIL'S STORY: SYMPTOMS IGNORED UNTIL A CRISIS OCCURS

The story of Janet and Phil Whiting, a couple married for over fifty years, is told by the physician Sherwin B. Nuland in his book *How We Die,* winner of the National Book Award.

In his boyhood in the 1930s, Nuland met the couple when Janet was just twenty and Phil twenty-two. An observation that the young Nuland made about this joyous couple, so different from his parents and other married people he knew, probably affected them deeply in later years, as Janet's denial about her husband's worsening condition made her life a disaster and kept him from diagnosis for years. Nuland writes, "I knew from personal observation that married people don't behave like this. If the Whitings expected things to work out, they would simply have to stop acting as though they were crazy about each other . . . To a great extent, they never did."

Years later, after four children and a successful career for Phil, Nuland bade a sad farewell to the couple as they moved from the New Haven, Connecticut, area to retirement in Florida. He was not aware that, even before the move, strange things had begun to happen, things noted by Janet only in retrospect, well after her husband had been diagnosed with probable Alzheimer's.

For one thing, Phil, possessed of an exceptionally

sharp and curious mind that he kept stimulated by the almost constant reading of nonfiction books, stopped reading entirely. He insisted that he and Janet be together all the time, telling her that he hadn't retired to be alone. Only after his condition had become much worse did she realize that he hadn't wanted her to go out by herself because he knew that something had started to happen to him, and that he was afraid to be left alone. Rarely angry when younger, he now seemed to have fairly frequent angry outbursts, which became full-blown tantrums before the move to Florida. He also so criticized their grown daughter Nancy when she visited that she would usually flee their condo in tears.

In Florida, incidents of confusion grew worse, with Phil always responding to them as if they were the other person's fault. For instance, he would go to the wrong barbershop for his haircuts, and become enraged that the barber did not recall their appointment. Angry incidents also increased.

Finally, something happened that would seemingly have been a loud call to action, but still Janet persisted in hoping and believing that nothing was wrong with her beloved Phil. They had a couple they hadn't seen for several years, the Warners, over for dinner. Phil had always been an excellent host, and this evening was no exception. The dinner went extremely well. Yet the next day, Phil remembered not an instant of it. Though frightened, Janet managed to convince herself that this very big memory problem was similar to the minor lapses she herself experienced from time to time.

However, a few weeks later, Phil began to accuse her of having taken a lover, and even worse, the so-called lover was a cousin of his who had been dead for years! Janet really became scared, but still did nothing *until about two years later.* By this time, Phil started to awaken in the night and angrily force her out of their bed, thinking she was his sister and yelling, "Since when does a sister sleep with her brother?" Always, by morning, he would forget the events had occurred. Using some excuse to get him to go to the doctor, she actually hoped that she would be told that nothing was wrong. Instead, he received a diagnosis of probable Alzheimer's.

At the time, in the mid-1980s, the Alzheimer's-specific drugs Aricept and Cognex were years in the future, and the disease was little understood by many, including physicians. Unfortunately, Phil's physician did not attempt to treat the symptoms he was experiencing, notably his hostility and aggression. Possibly as part of her denial about what was happening, not just to Phil but to her marriage and life in general, Janet did not seek the advice of another physician, nor did she turn to such support organizations as the Alzheimer's Association. She determined bravely, but somewhat unrealistically, to care for him at home all by herself until it was absolutely no longer possible. To this end she read a number of books, and found *The Thirty-six Hour Day* to be especially informative. In fact, a single sentence from that book finally ended her still-lingering hopes that, despite all that she had witnessed, and despite the doctor's opinion, what she was seeing in Phil was a natural part of aging. The sentence read: "Dementia is not the natural result of aging."

However, while Janet thought she had finally acknowledged to herself that her beloved husband was, indeed, ill, she still refused fully to cope with or prepare for the serious difficulties that come with a chronic disease like Alzheimer's. Her remaining denial about the true nature of the situation led to her resolute desire to care for Phil entirely by herself. Without a physician involved in treating Phil's symptoms, and without the information and comfort that a support organization would have provided—even lacking brief times of respite away from her constant duties—Janet's life with Phil got worse and worse.

From having read *The Thirty-six Hour Day,* Janet knew that sometimes the disease progressed to the point that those affected would throw things, or even strike their caregivers. Yet, until it actually happened, she hadn't believed it would, though Phil's worsening displays of anger and hostility were signs of such a possibility. Shortly before their fiftieth anniversary, Phil did not recognize her, and actually thought that she was a woman who had broken into the apartment to steal his wife's clothes. He pushed her around and threw things at her, then called their daughter Nancy to tell her what was going on. Mercifully, Nancy quickly figured out the situation, and asked Phil to let her speak with the thief, so she could also tell her to get out. As soon as Janet got on the phone, Nancy told her to leave the apartment immediately, and said she would phone the police. Janet hung up, and Phil himself grabbed the phone and called the police.

Later admitting it was a foolish decision, Janet stayed in the apartment, and Phil became more violent; she, too, then called the police. Three police cars arrived, as did a neighbor, who calmed Phil down. When next he looked at Janet, he recognized her—and excitedly told her about the woman who'd just been there trying to steal her clothes. One of the policemen coaxed Phil into his car and took him to a hospital, where he remained briefly before going into a nursing home.

And, indeed, the nursing home was a good setting for him, even better than the isolation of the apartment with Janet his only company. His gregarious good nature came to the fore early in his stay there, before the illness progressed further. In fact, he thought that he was in charge of a home of unwell people, people for whom he was responsible. Fully dressed, he would daily walk the wards, inquiring after each individual's welfare.

As Dr. Nuland points out in his discussion of Janet and Phil, everyone responds to a loved one's Alzheimer's in an individual way. Janet went to the nursing home daily, even volunteering in the physical therapy department. And while she briefly became involved in a support organization, she found that it was simply not for her at this point. She drew her emotional comfort from her grown children, and from some close, devoted friends. The children did not visit their father in the home, and she understood that they simply could not bear to see him in this state. They, realizing this fact about themselves, concentrated on taking care of their mother, insisting on periods of respite and giving her tremendous emotional support.

It's important to realize that Janet coped as well as she could at the time with the continuing decline of this single most important person in the world to her. The first signs of his illness appeared in the early 1980s, when many in the medical field did not recognize Alzheimer's as occurring primarily in the elderly; those with his symptoms would have been diagnosed with senile dementia, which was perceived as an unlucky part of natural aging for those who had it. By 1986, the time of his first doctor's appointment, more was understood, but the condition was still generally acknowledged as untreatable. The fact that Janet did not seek a doctor who would treat the symptoms of Phil's Alzheimer's came from this ignorance; the fact that she was blind to so much came from her deep love for her husband. Fortunately for those just showing symptoms nowadays, so much more is available, both medically and in terms of social services.

DIANA'S STORY: SYMPTOMS NOTED BY THE SUFFERER, BUT DENIED BY HER FIRST PHYSICIAN

All too often, the phenomenon of denial is not the exclusive province of sufferers and their families. This fact is strongly underlined in the book *Living in the Labyrinth*, Diana Friel McGowin's moving account of her experiences with the very rare early-onset Alzheimer's. Diana was first aware of having memory difficulties in her early forties. Since she had earlier had a minor stroke, she already had a relationship with a neurologist, a doctor who specializes in the care of the nervous system, which includes the brain.

Yet, much to her surprise, Diana's doctor did not take her concerns seriously. After all, to him, she was much too young to have an illness now generally associated with much older people, and he unfortunately turned out to be the type of doctor who gave more credence to general assumptions about illnesses than to his patient's own experiences. Further, he may also have been among those doctors, fortunately becoming more rare, who ascribe the complaints of female patients to psychological rather than physical causes. A doctor who thinks in this way does not deny that the patient indeed experiences the symptoms, but that they have a medical root.

At first Diana reluctantly accepted his opinion, though she grew increasingly worried at her mental lapses. Finally, in the wake of being lost in her car in her own neighborhood for four hours, she returned to the doctor and insisted on treatment. He merely prescribed mild tranquilizers and counseling with a psychologist. (As opposed to psychiatrists, who are medical doctors who specialize in the care of emotions and behavior, psychologists have completed the doctorate degree in the field of psychology.) On hearing her symptoms, however, the psychologist became concerned and conducted a number of tests that indicated the seriousness of Diana's condition. Yet when the psychologist refered her back to the neurologist for further testing and diagnosis, Diana was shocked by his response. The neurologist informed her that he was "not ready to take directions from an individual with only a degree in psychology." He insisted that she take an antidepressant, along with an additional dosage of the tranquilizer he initially prescribed, and repeated that she should undergo counseling.

Frightened by her experiences of disorientation and memory loss, Diana found this response unacceptable. She got a copy of her records, then phoned the local chapter of the Alzheimer's Association. She contacted the association not because she thought even for a moment that she might have Alzheimer's—after all, like her first neurologist, she assumed she was much too young—but because she believed it would be an excellent source to help her locate a doctor who would better deal with her concerns. A new doctor made no assumptions, and ensured that all the diagnostic tests were performed. Much to Diana's shock, she was finally informed of a diagnosis of probable Alzheimer's.

One would think that a person of Diana's age would simply collapse at such news, and see her productive years behind her once and for all. Yet while the news was, of course, quite an emotional blow, Diana's experience underlines the fact that the next stage of life *begins* with diagnosis. Knowing at last what disease she was facing, she got the right medical treatment and organized her legal and financial affairs. She also addressed a marriage that had been in trouble, and achieved a new closeness with her family. Further, she made incredible achievements in the public sphere, founding a society for early-onset Alzheimer's patients and wrote an influential book about her experiences, *Living in the Labyrinth*. Her experience of having to fight for a diagnosis was made available to even more people when major news organizations picked up her story and she was the subject of articles and featured on such national television shows as "20/20." In acting dynamically to get a diagnosis, and acting dynamically afterward, Diana not only improved her own life, but those of others.

TWO

WHAT EXACTLY IS ALZHEIMER'S?

AN ANCIENT DISEASE NAMED ONLY IN THIS CENTURY

Although the disease now known as Alzheimer's did not have a name until 1910, it is by no means new. Its symptoms have been noted throughout the centuries, starting with medical historians in the ancient world, and in literature as well as in life. The affliction suffered by King Lear, so movingly described by Shakespeare, was most likely Alzheimer's, as was the dementia that so marred the last years of the eighteenth-century writer Jonathan Swift.

Yet, as discussed by Sherwin Nuland, M.D., in his book *How We Die*, it took a nineteenth-century invention—the high-resolution microscope—combined with the skill of a turn-of-the-century German physician—Alois Alzheimer—to bring about an understanding of the illness as a distinct disease process.

DR. ALZHEIMER'S BREAKTHROUGH

Earlier physicians had, of course, worked with dementia patients and tried to understand the cause of their symptoms. A French physician, Jean Etienne Esquirol, had closely observed dementia patients, had performed autopsies on them, and had then remarked upon a number of ways that their brains differed from healthy ones. The high-resolution microscope, however, enabled Alzheimer to study brain tissue closely. He was then able to describe with much greater accuracy the changes in this tissue wrought by the disease that had killed one of his patients.

In examining the brain tissue of this woman, who had died in her fifties after experiencing several years of dementia, Alzheimer discovered what are now called amyloid or neuritic plaques and neurofibrillary tangles. He remarked upon the presence of some kind of harmful substance in the fibrils not present in healthy cells, which he perceived to be a product of the patient's own metabolism. (He was most likely describing the altered protein tau, found in neurofibrillary tangles. Another protein, beta amyloid, is now known to be in the neuritic plaques). Finally, he noted the degeneration or entire destruction of one quarter to one third of the cells in the cerebral cortex, the outer area of the brain, which involves such functions as reason, language, and conscious thought itself.

Alzheimer presented these findings in a 1907 paper, "On a Distinctive Disease of the Cerebral Cortex" (*"Uber eigenartige Erkrankung der Hirnrinde"*). His title revealed the news that he was describing a distinct disease process. And even now, it is the presence of a significant number of these plaques and tangles, discoverable only through autopsy, that is the primary sign that someone diagnosed with *probable* Alzheimer's in life truly had the disease.

Why was Alzheimer's thought to strike only those under sixty-five?

Dr. Emil Kraepelin, Alzheimer's mentor and a major figure in organic psychiatry, first called this disease process Alzheimer's disease, in a 1910 revision of his textbook. After stating his belief that the "clinical significance of Alzheimer's disease is still unclear," Kraepelin wrote that Alzheimer's findings "suggest that this condition deals with an especially severe form of senile dementia." He also pointed out, however, that the situation of the patient studied—she was hospitalized at fifty-one and died almost five years later—contradicted that conclusion. Importantly, he mentioned the words *senium praecox* (early senility) as a way of describing the condition, though he also wrote specifically that "this disease is more or less independent of age."

The uncertainty openly acknowledged by Kraepelin, a renowned expert in his field, led later authors to focus unduly on the term *senium praecox* and to discount his noting that the disease was "more or less independent of age."

Adding to the perception that Alzheimer's strikes the middle-aged (and sometimes those even younger), rather than the elderly, was the relative youth of those patients reported on in the medical journals. For, in the years after the publication of Alzheimer's paper and of Kraepelin's revised textbook, a number of physicians performed autopsies primarily on relatively youthful sufferers of dementia, usually noting the same findings in the brain tissue that Alzheimer had first described.

Not surprisingly, physicians tend to investigate unusual cases more thoroughly than run-of-the-mill ones. In situations where autopsies are not mandatory, they are most often performed on patients whose cases are perceived as interesting; in Nuland's words, "What could be more interesting than a young man with an old man's disease?"

By the end of the 1920s, therefore, medical literature showed a vast majority of Alzheimer's disease patients under the age of sixty.

Alzheimer's became seen as a relatively rare disease onsetting mainly in a patient's fifties, though occasionally it was noted in patients who were even younger. It was considered distinct from the dementia suffered by millions of older people, which was called simply "senile dementia."

This misconception continued for fifty years.

Was it important to realize that those under and over sixty-five have the same disease?

Certainly. In fact, it was a change that would affect millions of lives, and that would point to one of the major health crises of the twenty-first century.

The realization that there were not two distinct dementias, one appearing in relatively younger people and one seen among the elderly, gained credence in the late 1960s. A number of doctors recognized that both groups of patients had the same symptoms and the same post-mortem (after death) findings in the brain. In short, they had the same disease. This view was finally accepted by the medical establishment in the early 1970s.

It was a change that revolutionized the way Alzheimer's was seen.

No longer thought to be a rare disease barely worthy

of mention in medical schools—and hardly deserving of scarce research dollars—Alzheimer's became recognized as a leading health issue and, with the aging population, a public health time bomb. The patient population swelled to the millions, and their advocates, notably their families, amounted to millions more. And these millions wanted research dollars directed toward the disease.

What's happened as a result of Alzheimer's being seen as a major health issue?

Two Major Organizations Are Formed and Research Budgets Increase Drastically

Two major information and advocacy organizations were eventually formed in the wake of this realization of the true extent of Alzheimer's. They are the National Institute on Aging (the NIA) and the Alzheimer's Disease and Related Dementias Association (ADRDA—informally called the Alzheimer's Association).

By the beginning of the 1990s, monies allocated nationwide for research increased almost one thousand times over that available at the end of the 1970s.

Research has resulted in a better understanding of the disease process, which in turn results in the development of treatments. Specific ways that Alzheimer's affects the brain are discussed in more depth later in this chapter, and treatments of the disease itself, and of its behavioral symptoms, are mentioned here but presented more fully in Chapter Seven.

Cognex and Aricept, the First Two Drugs Developed Specifically for Alzheimer's

An important aspect of the Alzheimer's disease process is a serious decrease in the amount of the neurotransmitter acetylcholine, vital to memory.

In the 1990's, the FDA approved the first two drugs specifically developed to fight Alzheimer's. They are Cognex (tacrine) and Aricept (donepezil), and both treat Alzheimer's by addressing this decreased amount of acetylcholine. These drugs do not increase production of this neurotransmitter. They do, however, inhibit an enzyme called *cholinesterase*, which breaks down acetylcholine in the *synapse*, the gap between neurons that neurotransmitters must cross to transmit signals from one neuron to the next. Inhibiting cholinesterase enables acetylcholine to stay active in the synapse longer than it would have otherwise.

Recent studies have suggested an additional beneficial effect of both drugs. At higher doses, they may decrease abnormal accumulation of amyloid, a protein implicated in the disease process.

Approved a few years later than Cognex, Aricept is easier to take (once a day rather than four times), and it does not seem to inflame the liver as Cognex may in some people. As they do with all drugs, people react differently to these two. While some people show only minor improvement, others have benefitted tremendously from their use.

Drugs Developed for Other Illnesses That May Be Useful in Treating Alzheimer's

Though Cognex and Aricept were the first drugs developed specifically to treat Alzheimer's, researchers and clinicians have discovered that the *off-label* use of several already existing drugs can be effective against various aspects of the disease process (the term off-label use means using drugs to treat one disease when they've been approved by the FDA for another disease or diseases.) They include nicotine, estrogen, and antihypertensive drugs (developed to treat high blood pressure).

A number of these off-label drugs are currently being tested in *double-blind, placebo-controlled protocols*, the most rigorous and informative kind of study, to more clearly establish just how effective they are against Alzheimer's.

Drugs That Treat the Behaviorial Symptoms of Alzheimer's

Researchers and clinicians have realized as well that a number of the symptoms of Alzheimer's, including severe agitation and anxiety, depression, and insomnia, can also be treated by existing drugs. Among these drugs are *neuroleptics* such as Haldol and Mellaril, which treat severe agitation and psychotic symptoms, such as hallucinations; antidepressants such as Prozac and Tofranil; and sleeping medications such as Restoril and Ambien.

Non-drug Substances Found to be Effective Against Alzheimer's

Antioxidant vitamins such as E and C and Coenzyme Q-10, and herbs such as ginkgo biloba, an extract from the leaf of the ginkgo tree, have also been found to help some people with Alzheimer's. And

American medicine, which seemed to be looking down on these kinds of treatments when not ignoring them entirely, has become more open to investigating their usefulness in rigorous *protocols*, carefully controlled drug studies.

Other Coping Techniques Discovered and Refined

A variety of therapies and activities have been developed to give the Alzheimer's patient a greater sense of confidence, safety and comfort. By calming the patient, they also help caregivers in their day-to-day coping. They include *orientation therapy* and a technique called *reminiscing*. These are discussed in Chapter Eight.

What is the current state of research?

Almost every day seems to herald the discovery of yet another piece in the puzzle that is Alzheimer's—studies investigating and further establishing beneficial effects of herbs such as ginkgo biloba, or of drugs such as estrogen, or of antioxidants such as vitamin E, as well as promising findings in the quest to understand the disease on a genetic level.

Genetic research may, indeed, one day lead to therapies that cure Alzheimer's. Yet it is most important right now for further revealing the metabolic steps of the disease process. This knowledge is our strongest hope for better treatments, among them more drug and nutritional therapies that can intervene in those steps.

THE DISEASE PROCESS CALLED ALZHEIMER'S— WHAT IS NOW KNOWN ABOUT IT

A Disease of the Central Nervous System

Alzheimer's is a progressive, degenerative disease of the central nervous system; such diseases are marked by a decay in the structure of tissue and its function, a decay that becomes worse over time. You've probably heard of other diseases of this type, among them Parkinson's disease, Huntington's disease and Lou Gehrig's disease (ALS). You probably haven't yet heard of others, among them Pick's disease and primary progressive aphasia. You'll be reading about these, and other causes of dementia, in Chapter Three.

As you read in Chapter One, the onset of Alzheimer's is so gradual and slow that it is difficult for those around the ill person even to notice changes until several years after the disease process has begun. Most people are not diagnosed for five to seven years after they first show symptoms.

And the symptoms of Alzheimer's are among the most heartrending of any disease—forgetting where you are, forgetting loved ones, finally forgetting your very self. The central nervous system must be powerful indeed, if a disease that affects it, so affects us.

The Central Nervous System— A Personal Command Center

Made up of the brain and the spinal cord, the *central nervous system* is the main division of the nervous system in the body. The others are the *autonomic nervous system* and the *peripheral nervous system*. These are made up of the motor and sensory nerves outside of the brain and spinal cord.

By directing commands to the rest of the body through nerve fibers that run through the spinal cord, the brain controls vital bodily functions and sensations. They include the ones that ensure our daily survival, maintaining us as physical beings—among them sleep, muscle movement, thirst, and hunger. And, by controlling sexual activity, the brain also ensures our survival as a species.

Our Brains, Ourselves

Yet the brain also controls much more subtle functions and sensations. Consider, a moment, those inborn, seemingly unchangeable factors that make up our individual personalities. You know, the ones that people have come to count on in us:

They may be generosity, or a quick wit, or a touch of sarcasm, or a love of animals:

They may be the interests that express our personalities—spending long hours alone, reveling in gardening, playing the piano, or reading big, fat novels; or devoting spare hours to social pursuits, such as dancing, card games or gossipy get-togethers over coffee (or a few beers).

They may even be matters of physical taste and habit that have come to be seen as part of our personalities, such as a lifelong aversion to very sweet desserts, or a firm belief in—and practice of—an "early to bed, early to rise" approach to sleep.

All these qualities that, added up, make up the individual self are not in reality constant and never changing; they depend on the healthy functioning of the brain.

THE TWO REGIONS OF THE BRAIN MOST AFFECTED BY ALZHEIMER'S

Alzheimer's affects first the *hippocampus,* then the *cerebral cortex,* in a number of ways. In reading about these two regions you'll better understand why damage to them produces the symptoms associated with Alzheimer's.

The Hippocampus

While the very earliest signs of Alzheimer's are now known to be found in a small region called the *entorhinal cortex,* deep within the brain, the nearby hippocampus is the first to be strongly affected by the disease. It is where memories are literally made, from our earliest recollections to information learned but a minute ago. And memories are not solely made in the hippocampus, but stored there as well, waiting to respond to the signal that we need to retrieve them (as all of us age, the retrieval process can become slower and slower). It is fitting, then, that this center of memory formation and storage is located deep within the brain, since it holds the core of our individual identities.

The Cerebral Cortex

A thin layer of gray matter on the surface of the brain, the cerebral cortex is associated with such higher functions as language, reason, and judgment. Yet these vital aspects of the self are not the only functions associated with this region of the brain.

Over two hundred distinct areas of the cerebral cortex have been described by researchers, as well as almost fifty different functions. A range of activities such as stomach functions and behavioral reactions are directed by the cerebral cortex. The area controlling motor function is found here, and not just those voluntary motions we consciously control and use to perform a wide variety of actions. Stimulation of the frontal areas of the cerebral cortex has been shown to affect involuntary activities, from widening of the pupils to such basic functions as circulation and breathing.

Simply put, damage to the cerebral cortex is devastating.

WHAT ALZHEIMER'S DOES TO THE BRAIN

Related Effects Not Yet Fully Understood

Following is a list of a number of changes in the brain noted in Alzheimer's; each is discussed in more detail right after the list. A major goal of research is to better understand these changes—how they occur, how they influence each other, and, ultimately, how they can be affected, or even prevented.

- A decrease in the amount of the neurotransmitter acetylcholine.
- The formation of amyloid, or neuritic, plaques outside neurons, and of neurofibrillary tangles inside neurons.
- Damage to and the death of many neurons, notably *cholinergic neurons*, which are vital to the production of acetylcholine.
- Problems in the process called *glucose metabolism*.

- Damage to the *mitochondria*. Components of all cells, they are involved in the production of energy.

A Decreased Amount of a Vital Brain Chemical

Most of us experience a certain decrease in acetyl-choline as we age; it's probably a major factor in age-related cognitive decline, the mild forgetting that sooner or later starts to plague us.

A reason for this decrease is the damage to and death of cholinergic neurons, which produce *acetylcholine*. Many more cholinergic neurons are damaged and destroyed in those who develop Alzheimer's than those who do not. People with Alzheimer's, therefore, experience a much greater decrease in acetylcholine than normal, so communication within their brains is much more strongly affected.

As discussed previously, the drugs Cognex and Aricept treat Alzheimer's by keeping acetylcholine active in the synapse longer than it would be without their use.

Amyloid or Neuritic Plaques and Neurofibrillary Tangles

As Alzheimer's progresses and more and more amyloid or neuritic plaques form outside neurons and neurofibrillary tangles form within them, the neurons themselves are damaged and even die. While this process is not fully understood, it is believed that several factors damage and destroy neurons:

1. The neuritic plaques and neurofibrillary tangles crowd out the neurons.

2. The plaques and tangles cause inflammation that damages and destroys neurons.
3. The tangles prevent nutrients from flowing through the neurons, starving them.
4. Beta amyloid, the main component of the plaques, may in itself be toxic to neurons.

TWO PROTEINS THAT ARE CRUCIAL—AND UNSOLVED—PIECES OF THE ALZHEIMER'S PUZZLE

Beta Amyloid

Beta amyloid is in fact not a protein but a protein fragment, and the amyloid or neuritic plaques that form outside of neurons are important because they contain a-beta. Researchers have studied beta amyloid intently, and some groundbreaking information has been the result. Kenneth Davis, M.D., a leading researcher at New York's Mount Sinai Medical School, views the discovery that a-beta is the component of amyloid in the plaques as one of the most important of recent years. It may indeed lead to the type of effective treatments of Alzheimer's that researchers have long sought.

The beta amyloid protein is a string of about forty *amino acids*, compounds vital to the formation of proteins. It is formed when enzymes called proteases snip it from a larger protein called *amyloid precursor protein*, or APP, when APP protrudes through the neuron *membrane*, or the cell wall. The action of a number of these enzymes, called *alpha-, beta-,* and *gamma-secretases,* determines if the type of amyloid produced is the plaque-forming beta amyloid.

For instance, theoretically, when APP and the component that can become beta amyloid are snipped apart by alpha-secretase, amyloid is formed, but amyloid plaques do not result because there is no beta amyloid to form them. However, if either beta-secretase or gamma-secretase snips the fragment from APP, the beta amyloid molecule is produced. This molecule can form into the amyloid found in plaques.

Is it possible to intervene in the production of beta amyloid and thereby prevent the formation of the amyloid plaques? Researchers are seeking a way to alter the processing of APP into beta amyloid, and have investigated the possibility of inhibiting beta- and gamma-secretase, or trying to enhance alpha-secretase. Since, however, any molecule that affects these proteases would affect a number of processes in addition to amyloid production, that approach is not workable.

Other approaches have been studied. Perhaps it will eventually be possible simply to stop beta amyloid's aggregating into plaques, rather than stopping its production. As noted earlier in the chapter, recent studies have shown that in higher doses, both Cognex and Aricept may be antiaggregating agents.

In the quest for treatments researchers are also investigating the following questions:

1. Does beta amyloid reduce the amount of choline in neurons, thereby reducing the amount of acetylcholine? Does it in fact contribute to, or even cause, the death of cholinergic neurons?
2. In addition to forming plaques, does some of the beta amyloid break into fragments, thereby releasing *free radicals*, molecules that damage and even destroy cells?

3. Beta amyloid has been shown to form tiny channels in neuron membranes. Do these channels allow a lethal overdose of calcium into neurons?

4. What is the connection between beta amyloid and *apolipoprotein* (*apoE*), in particular the apoE produced by the *allele*, or form, of the apoE gene known as *apoE4*? The apoE4 protein binds tightly and insolubly with beta amyloid, while the *apoE3* protein, produced by the apoE3 allele, does not.

5. Does the *apoE2* protein actually help guard against Alzheimer's? If so, how can this protective function be adapted for a treatment? (More information about the genetics of Alzheimer's is discussed later in the chapter.)

Altered Tau

Further questions focus on this protein, a major component of the tangles found within the neurons.

The function of tau was revealed by researchers in the late 1980s. In a healthy neuron, internal, train-track-like structures called *microtubules* carry nutrients from the cell body to the end of the *axon,* the long structure leading away from the neuron toward the *dendrites* of nearby neurons. Tau forms the railroad ties, as it were, of these structures.

In the disease process of Alzheimer's, however, neurofibrillary tangles are formed when an altered version of tau twists the microtubules into *paired helical filaments*, which look like two threads wrapped around each other.

These misshapen microtubules cannot carry nutrients the length of the neuron, from the body through the axons. The neuron starves.

The Death of Cholinergic Neurons

You have already read that cholinergic neurons, vital to the production of acetylcholine, die off in tremendous numbers during the Alzheimer's disease process. As discussed in the previous section, amyloid plaques and neurofibrillary tangles are involved in the death of these neurons in several ways, including the following:

1. The abnormal accumulation of beta amyloid into plaques crowds out these neurons, and causes inflammation that also damages them.
2. The beta amyloid in the plaques is in itself toxic to the neurons.
3. The beta amyloid protein fragment can break, releasing free radicals that damage the neurons in a number of ways. One way discussed in a following section is by damaging the mitochondria, which are responsible for metabolizing glucose and oxygen to provide energy for the neurons.
4. The neurofibrillary tangles prevent the flow of nutrients through the neurons, thereby starving them.
5. Beta amyloid creates tiny channels in the membrane of the neuron, possibly allowing uncontrolled, potentially fatal amounts of calcium into the neurons.
6. Beta amyloid may also disrupt potassium channels, which would also affect calcium levels in the neurons.

These effects can seem almost overwhelming. However, progress is being made in fighting the death of cholinergic neurons. Kenneth Davis, M.D., finds tremendous promise in an unexpected result in the use of Cognex and Aricept, the drugs that inhibit cholinesterase, and allow acetylcholine more time to deliver messages from one neuron to another. Something in the stimulation of cholinergic activity seems to alter the way APP is processed; it decreases the production of beta amyloid, the plaque-forming protein, and increases the production of peptides that do not produce amyloid. Cognex and Aricept can help certain Alzheimer's patients in more ways than one.

Another factor pertaining to the health of cholinergic neurons has proven beneficial to many Alzheimer's patients. It is a basic, seemingly simple factor, but one that tends to get overlooked in a fast-paced, fat-phobic world that favors convenience in meal preparation and slenderness in body type. It is nutrition.

Fat-related substances such as estrogen, vitamin E, and omega-3 fatty acids nourish cholinergic neurons; their use is being studied further. Depletion of estrogen in menopause seems to contribute to the development of Alzheimer's in some women, since studies have shown that women who take estrogen replacement therapy do not develop Alzheimer's at the rate of those who don't take such therapy. Deficiencies in vitamin E and omega-3 fatty acids also seem to harm these neurons.

Glucose Metabolism

As you'll read in the next section, *glucose,* or sugar, is combined with oxygen in the mitochondria of a cell to lead to the production of the energy that allows the cell to carry out its function. Known as glucose metabolism, this process is somehow connected to Alzheimer's disease, though it is not yet understood exactly how.

Researchers have been better able to study this process due to the fairly recent development of a scanner called the *PET scan* (PET is short for *positron emission tomography*), which enables researchers to track the flow of glucose and oxygen molecules within the brain. Those areas with glucose and oxygen in the bloodstream are producing energy and are therefore active. As the disease progresses, more and more areas of the brain do not show the presence of glucose and oxygen; those areas have become inactive.

Glucose metabolism declines dramatically as neurons are damaged and eventually die. However, it is not known if this decline is due to the state of the neurons, or if a problem with the glucose metabolism process itself contributes to it. During the process glucose molecules are carried by *capillaries* past neurons; on their way they are captured by molecules whose function is to take glucose molecules from the capillaries and move them into neurons.

These transporter molecules come in several forms. In the cerebral cortex of Alzheimer's patients there are lower levels of two forms of them (GLUT1 and GLUT2). These lower levels may account for the reduction of glucose metabolism in this region of the brain. However, the state of the capillaries themselves could contribute to the reduction of glucose levels in neurons; if capillary walls have thickened due to deposits of cholesterol or other substances, the flow of glucose molecules could be affected.

Once they reach the inside of the neuron, glucose molecules are taken to the mitochondria, where they will undergo the process that turns them into energy. And in the mitochondria is yet another clue to the Alzheimer's puzzle.

Damage to Mitochondria

Mitochondria are vital to all the cells in the body, since they put glucose and oxygen together to produce *adenosine triphosphate* (ATP), a chemical vital in energizing cells. The genes in the mitochondria are responsible for the production of thirteen proteins, many of which are used in the formation of ATP. If any of these genes are faulty, resulting in problems in ATP formation, the cells that need ATP for energy cannot perform their functions. And neurons need a lot of energy to carry out their functions.

Mitochondria are unusual in that they contain genetic material from the mother alone. Nonmitochondrial DNA, inherited from both parents, is in the cell nucleus and is protected by proteins called *histones*. Mitochondria lie outside the nucleus of the cell and their DNA has no such protection. It is much easier for it to be damaged.

A research team led by Davis Parker, M.D., of the University of Virginia, a neurologist, investigated the effect of mutated mitochondrial DNA. By implanting mitochondria with mutant DNA into nerve cells from which all mitochondrial DNA, but not nuclear DNA, had been removed, the researchers found that these cells produce a less efficient form of one of the proteins needed to produce ATP than cells with nondamaged mitochondria. Another important finding is that the cells also tended to contain many more free radicals than those with healthy mitochondrial DNA.

Such problems occurring in the mitochondria of cholinergic neurons could therefore lie behind the damage to those cells and the decrease in their production of acetylcholine.

FREE RADICALS—THE BAD BOYS BEHIND AGING

The term free radical is actually short for *oxygen free radical molecule*. Free radicals are formed during the process of metabolism, which is the converting of food into energy.

Unlike other oxygen molecules, these renegade molecules have an uneven number of electrons in their outer shell, meaning that one of the electrons is not paired. It can latch onto another molecule—which free radicals do eagerly, as they are highly reactive. And the molecules that free radicals latch on to can be as important as those in DNA or cell membranes. Free radicals are capable of causing considerable damage since their latching onto other molecules sets off chemical reactions that can be harmful to cells.

Free radicals have been implicated in a number of steps in the Alzheimer's disease process, as well as in diseases ranging from cancer to glaucoma. While they can cause cell damage in general, they have specific connections to Alzheimer's. They may damage the DNA of mitochondria and they may damage *phospholipids,* the fat molecules in the membranes of neurons. Damage to the membrane means that the cell cannot control amounts of substances that enter it, including potentially fatal ones such as calcium.

And of course, free radicals are involved in the very process of aging itself whether or not a person has Alzheimer's.

There are some defenses against free radicals,

however, notably the antioxidant vitamins, vitamin E and vitamin C. Other substances shown to be helpful to Alzheimer's patients, such as ginkgo biloba, are believed to have antioxidant properties.

THE GENETIC CONNECTION

What Genes Do

Genes enable cells to express (to carry out) their particular function, most often the production of proteins such as hormones and enzymes. These proteins and other substances direct the functioning of the body.

The basic element of living tissue, cells are made up of a *nucleus* (basically, the "brain" of that particular cell), and of cytoplasm (the "body" of the cell). The nucleus is itself comprised of the *nucleolus*, which contains *RNA (ribonucleic acid)*, which carries gene data from the nucleus to the *cytoplasm* and *chromatin granules*, which contain protein and *DNA (deoxyribonucleic acid*, which contains genetic information).

Chromosomes—Where Genes Are Located

Within the nucleus of the cell are *chromosomes*, threadlike structures made up of a double strand of twisted DNA. It is on these strands that the genes are located.

Four chemicals or bases, arranged in sequences, make up each gene. Just as each gene has a different sequence of bases, each gene directs the manufacture of a different protein. Even a slight defect in a gene can seriously affect its particular function, the code for the proteins for which it, and it alone, is responsible.

A faulty protein can, in turn, lead to the malfunction of a cell, and, eventually, to disease.

The Chromosomes Connected to Alzheimer's

Alzheimer's has so far been linked to four chromosomes, numbers 1, 14, 19, and 21. Late-onset Alzheimer's, the most common type, is connected to chromosome 19, for which the defective gene has been found. It is the gene for apolipoproteinE (apoE). ApoE4, one form (or *allele*) of this gene, greatly increases the risk of disease, especially when inherited from both parents.

Note that *risk* is increased; having this form of the gene does not guarantee that a person will get Alzheimer's, nor does not having it mean that a person won't develop the disease. This lack of complete information is one of the issues that complicates the question of whether genetic testing should be sought, a topic discussed in Chapter Nine.

THREE

IT ISN'T ALWAYS ALZHEIMER'S —
OTHER CAUSES OF DEMENTIA

While Alzheimer's is the single most common cause of dementia, it is not the only one. Quite a range of diagnoses were finalized in just one typical week at the Department of Neurology and Neuroscience at the New York Hospital/Cornell University Medical College. Such major urban centers are often referred cases that are difficult to diagnose by individual doctors and by other centers.

Besides Alzheimer's, dementia was determined to be caused by:

1. The relatively rare Pick's disease.
2. The relatively rare primary progressive aphasia.
3. Depression (a condition known as pseudodementia).
4. Parkinson's disease.
5. HIV infection.
6. Vascular dementia (formerly called *multi-infarct dementia*, or MID)—the second most common cause of dementia after Alzheimer's.

In a typical week at a center based at a suburban hospital, several cases of Alzheimer's and vascular dementia were finalized. In addition to these, two cases were diagnosed not as dementia but as amnestic disorders (involving memory problems only and not other problems with thinking). Three other patients had tested positive for Lyme disease, though they had not yet completed the diagnostic process.

A NUMBER OF CAUSES MAY UNDERLIE DEMENTIA

Dementia can result from certain diseases or conditions, as well as from exposure to toxic metals and from longterm use of substances as prescription medications and alcohol. Remember that more than one cause can be behind a particular person's dementia. This is called a *mixed dementia,* and the most common one is that of Alzheimer's combined with vascular dementia. The various causes are listed below, then the first three are detailed later in the chapter.

The Causes of Dementia

1. *Degenerative disorders of the central nervous system*—these include Alzheimer's disease, Parkinson's disease, and Huntington's disease. The first two combined affect over five million individuals, not to mention their millions of relatives whose lives are also affected.
2. *Viral, bacterial, and other infections*—these include meningitis, syphilis, Lyme disease, encephalitis, and HIV. Dementia can be a longterm consequence of these infections.

3. *Cerebrovascular disorders*—these include vascular dementia (formerly known as multi-infarct dementia) and inflammatory diseases of blood vessels, including lupus (systemic lupus erythematosus).
4. *Medications*—chronic use of certain medications (using medications over a lengthy period of time) can cause confusion and memory loss. Among the many medications that can cause confusion and memory loss are those frequently used to treat older people:

Some Drugs that Impair Cognition

Type of Drug	Generic Name	Brand Name
antiarrhythmic drugs	quinidine sulfate/ gluconate	Quinidex
antibiotics	cephalexin	Keflex, others
	ciprofloxacin	Cipro
	metronidazole	Flagyl
antidepressant drugs	amitriptyline	Elavil, etc.
	doxepin	Sinequan, Adapin
	imipramine	Tofranil, etc.
anticonvulsant drugs	carbamazeoine	Tegretol
	phenytoin	Dilantin
	valproic acid/ divalproex sodium	Depakene, Depakote

antihistamines	chlorpheniramine	Chlor-Trimeton
	diphenhydramine	Benadryl, Tylenol PM, Excedrin PM
	phenylpropanolamine HCI	several OTC brands
	pseudoephedrine HCI/sulfate	Sudafed, Actifed
antinauseant drugs	hydroxyzine HCI	Atarax, Vistaril
	meclizine	Antivert, others
	metoclopramide	Reglan, etc.
	prochlorperazine	Compazine
antipsychotic drugs	chlorpromazine	Thorazine
	perphenazine	Trilafon
	thioridazine	Mellaril
	triflluoperazine	Stelazine
cardiac drugs	propranolol	Inderal
	timolol	Timoptic, Blocadren
drugs used in Parkinson's	benztropine mesylate	Cogentin Artane,
	trihexyphenidyl	Trihexy-2

narcotic analgesics	codeine sulfate/ phosphate	Tylenol with Codeine
	hydrocodone	Vicodin
	meperidine	Demerol
	oxycodone	Percodan
	propoxyphene	Darvon
sedatives	alprazolam	Xanax
	chlordiazepoxide	Librium, etc.
	diazepam	Valium
	flurazepam	Dalmane
	lorazepam	Ativan
	triazolam	Halcion

AN IMPORTANT NOTE: NEVER STOP TAK-ING ANY DRUGS ON YOUR OWN.

5. *Toxins*—among these are:
   Alcohol (long-term abuse)
   Anesthesia (in excessive amounts or through numerous administrations)
   Heavy metals (arsenic, bismuth, gold [during therapy for arthritis], lead, manganese, mercury)
   Industrial agents (carbon disulfide, carbon mon-
   oxide, organophosphates, toluene, trichloroeth-
   ylene)
6. *Trauma to the head*—dementia can be caused by
   injury to the brain due to repeated blows to the head
   (boxing can produce the aptly named *dementia
   pugilistica*) or by a single severe blow, such as that
   which might be incurred by falling from a height,
   say, off a ladder. (Such an accident could result in
   a *subdural hematoma*, a pooling of blood below the

dura of the brain.) Blows leading to unconscious-
ness of five minutes or more, even when they don't
cause a subdural hematoma, can also result in dementia years down the road due to the amount of
the protein amyloid the brain produces in response
to this type of injury. (Amyloid is discussed in detail in Chapter Two.)

7. *Nutritional deficiencies*—insufficient amounts of
folic acid, niacin, thiamine, and vitamin B_{12} can
cause dementia. Years of chronic alcoholism can
lead to nutritional deficiencies; very heavy drinkers
simply don't eat enough, or properly. Other conditions reflecting a nutritional deficiency include re-
current hypoglycemia (low glucose) and pernicious
anemia, a B_{12} deficiency, in which the symptoms
that would progress to eventual dementia begin in
middle age. Classic signs of pernicious anemia are
a lack of stature, pale skin, premature graying of
the hair, and the sensation of pins and needles.

8. *Endocrine and metabolic disorders*—among these
are hypothyroidism, which may be reversible, Ad-
dison's disease, and Cushing's syndrome (in which
the most common cause of mental impairment is
the use of steroids in high doses over time).

9. *Lesions to the brain*—a lesion is defined as a
wound, injury, or other destructive change in body
tissue. The lesions we think of most commonly in
connection with the brain are tumors, both benign
(noncancerous) and malignant (cancerous).

10. *Miscellaneous neurological conditions*—these include normal-pressure hydrocephalus (which may
account for up to one quarter of reversible dementias), multiple sclerosis, and epilesy.

11. *Affective disorders*—*affect* is the term used by phy-

sicians to refer to mood. The major affective disorder pertaining to dementia is depression, which can produce a condition known as *pseudodementia*. This condition is almost entirely reversible.

DEGENERATIVE DISORDERS OF THE CENTRAL NERVOUS SYSTEM

As discussed in Chapter Two, a progressive, degenerative disease is marked by a decay in the structure of tissue and its function.

The more common degenerative disorders of the central nervous system are Alzheimer's disease, Parkinson's disease, and Huntington's disease. There is strong evidence of another common central nervous system disorder, *diffuse Lewy body disease*. (The presence of Lewy bodies—spherical, white-blood-cell-filled bodies found in brain cells—has, until recently, been seen as part of Parkinson's; we now think it may be a subtype of Alzheimer's or even a separate disorder.)

Other more rare diseases include *amyotrophic lateral sclerosis* (ALS), also known as Lou Gehrig's disease, *frontal lobe degeneration of the non-Alzheimer's type,* primary progressive aphasia, and Pick's disease.

The medical text *Dementia*, edited by Peter J. Whitehouse, M.D., Ph.D, gives the following rates of prevalence for Alzheimer's and Parkinson's.

Alzheimer's. Out of the total population, estimates range from approximately 2 to 5 percent of those sixty-five and over. (In its rarer forms, Alzheimer's can onset earlier.) A study of East Boston residents published in the *Journal of the American Medical Association* in 1989 showed 3 percent of those aged sixty-five to seventy-four as having Alzheimer's, 18.7 percent of those seventy-five to eighty-four as being affected, and 47 percent of those over eighty-four. Millions of people are affected nationwide and the cost to society is in the billions of dollars.

These percentages reflect prevalence in the population as a whole. Yet when only those with dementia are considered, the percentage of those with Alzheimer's rises sharply. Diagnostic centers report anywhere from about 55 to about 70 percent of dementia cases as being due to Alzheimer's. For instance, the Framingham Study (results published in *Neurology* in January of 1992) reported 56 percent of demented individuals as being diagnosed with Alzheimer's alone, with an additional 12 percent having multiple causes. (Alzheimer's is frequently a factor in these mixed dementias.)

Parkinson's. About 1 percent of the U.S. population over fifty is believed to have Parkinson's, or approximately 2.5 million people. Later on in the disease many suffer from dementia.

The other central nervous system disorders affect a far smaller percentage of people. Still, with a population the size of that of the U.S., that can mean anywhere from tens to hundreds of thousands of people.

VIRAL, BACTERIAL, AND OTHER INFECTIONS

An infection is the invasion of the body by microorganisms (commonly known as germs) that then reproduce and multiply. They cause disease by injuring cells or by germ-antibody reaction in the cells.

A viral infection is caused by the transfer of the tiny organisms known as viruses from one body to another.

(Viruses can live only in the cells of another animal.) These transfers occur through breaks in the skin, through the intestines if a virus has been ingested, through an airborne virus being breathed in, through blood transfusions, and through unprotected sex.

Viruses have been in the news of late, and are among the star players in the book and television film *And the Band Played On*, in *The New Yorker* article that was expanded into the book *The Hot Zone*, and in the film *Outbreak*.

Yet viruses aren't the only cause of infections. While, for instance, viruses can cause some forms of meningitis, the most common causes of meningitis are bacteria, tiny, one-celled animals. Bacterial infections are treated with antibiotics.

We don't yet know if infections may be involved in the onset of such varied diseases as Alzheimer's and multiple sclerosis. (Remember how surprised we all were to learn that gastrointestinal ulcers might be caused by bacteria and could be treated with antibiotics?) For instance, since not all those who have the apoE4 gene develop Alzheimer's, perhaps an infectious agent triggers the gene in those who do.

A range of infections can have dementia as a symptom. They include Creutzfeldt-Jakob disease, encephalitis, HIV, Lyme disease, meningitis, and syphilis. While most of us tend to associate dementia with the advanced stage of a disease, if an infection has first affected the brain, dementia could well be the presenting symptom (the symptom that causes someone to seek medical help in the first place). Memory diagnostic centers at rare times encounter dementia as the first noticeable symptom of both AIDS (HIV) and Lyme disease.

THE VASCULAR DEMENTIAS: MULTI-INFARCT DEMENTIA AND OTHER CEREBROVASCULAR DEMENTIAS

Cerebrovascular disorders are those affecting the flow of blood to and within the brain. An unimpeded cerebral blood flow (CBF) is vital to the brain's full functioning, since blood carries oxygen and other vital nutrients. Though the brain is only about 2 percent of body weight, it takes 20 percent of cardiac output, fully ten times what its weight alone would merit. Dementias caused by a problem in CBF are called vascular dementias.

The most common vascular dementia is multi-infarct dementia (MID). It is currently believed to be the second most common single cause of dementia after Alzheimer's. The most common mixed dementia—the 10 percent of cases in which a person's dementia results from more than one cause—is that of Alzheimer's combined with MID.

MID results from small strokes, called infarctions. Almost without exception it is found in people with hypertension (high blood pressure) or cardiac arrythymias (abnormal beating of the heart). Infarctions are areas of tissues that have died and then decayed because blood can no longer reach them so the oxygen that was nourishing them was cut off. Infarctions occur due to the occluding (the blocking) of blood vessels. These blockages result from the formation of *thrombi* and *emboli*, medical terms for collections of cholesterol, other lipids (fats), and other matter in the blood vessels.

Different parts of the brain will be affected in each person with MID, depending on where the infarcts take place, since different parts of the brain have different functions. As tissues in different areas die off, what those areas control will be affected. At first MID has a "steplike" progression of symptoms. Someone will seem to be fine, then one day his speech will be mildly slurred. Nothing else may happen for a few months, when another problem will surface, such as difficulties with short-term memory. As it progresses, MID loses this steplike onset, looking more like Alzheimer's.

The risk factors for MID in general are those for cardiovascular disease, first and foremost hypertension. Other risk factors are smoking, obesity, being overweight if not obese, and lack of exercise; all of these lead to hypertension. High levels of cholesterol and triglycerides are also risk factors. Usually, MID first appears in those sixty to seventy-five years of age, due to the fact that it takes until one is sixty for the vascular damage to be severe enough to affect someone, and anyone with high enough risk factors to develop the condition is likely to have suffered a fatal stroke or heart attack by the age of seventy-five.

When you consider the symptoms that will eventually result in someone with MID going (or being taken) to a doctor for diagnosis, you can see how important it is to have a thorough exam by a diagnostician experienced in this area. (In Chapter Four we show you how to locate such a person.) Vascular dementia and Alzheimer's share a number of symptoms, many of which are too often incorrectly perceived as "natural" aspects of aging. These are discussed in detail in Chapter One, and are seen in the diagnostic charts in the Appendix.

A striking feature of vascular dementia is impaired emotional control. A sufferer can become moved to tears very easily, no matter how stoic he may have been in earlier years. Laughter in a situation that definitely does not call for it is another example of this impairment. Of course, these inappropriate expressions of emotion can lead to a great deal of embarrassment.

What features most distinguish MID from Alzheimer's? The initial steplike nature of the onset, which often allows the patient and family to point specifically to the beginning of noticeable symptoms (though in retrospect, they may realize that some more subtle symptoms actually were present earlier). Also, while frequently experiencing the same difficulties with short-term memory as those with Alzheimer's, MID patients usually do not confabulate to cover these deficiencies, while someone with Alzheimer's often will (to *confabulate* is to invent detailed, convincing events intended to "cover" the memory loss). Someone with MID will be, for example, greatly embarrassed that he cannot remember a grown child's phone number, but will admit to the deficit, while someone with Alzheimer's may blithely make up a number without missing a beat. (Note: Confabulation is a defense mechanism common not solely to Alzheimer's, but to those with head injuries, those suffering from lead poisoning, and some chronic alcoholics who suffer from a dementia called Korsakoff's psychosis.)

Due to symptoms shared by Alzheimer's and other dementias, neuroimaging—PET and SPECT scans, CT scans and MRIs—is especially helpful in the differential diagnosis of vascular dementia. You'll read more about these in Chapter Six.

Other vascular dementias include:

Subdural hematoma. *Hematoma* is the medical term for bruise, a pooling of blood that has escaped from the vessels and has become trapped in between the tissues of the skin or in an organ. Dura mater is the outermost of the three membranes surrounding the brain (the dura mater encephali) and spinal cord (the dura mater spinalis). A *subdural hematoma*, then, is a pooling of blood trapped below the dura mater of the skull. These arise from a hard blow to the head (they are also mentioned under the category of trauma to the head).

An *acute* subdural (an abrupt onset of severe confusion) hematoma has symptoms more like those of delirium than dementia, which will occur from a few days until about two weeks after the injury.

A *chronic* subdural hematoma, which may have dementia as a symptom, develops more slowly over time, from many weeks to months after the injury.

A clinical exam may determine the presence of a subdural hematoma through neurologic findings such as weakness in one side of the body and visual difficulties. A CT or MRI scan is used to diagnose possible structural lesions such as subdural hematoma. It's important to relieve the pressure that the hematoma creates in the brain. Treatment could include the use of steroids to decrease swelling and inflammation or even surgery, including the burr hole procedure, the drilling of holes in the skull to remove the hematoma and relieve the pressure it creates.

Binswanger's disease. Also referred to as *subcortical arteriosclerotic encephalopathy*, it is marked by changes in the white matter of the brain, revealed in autopsy—enlarged lateral ventricles (normal spaces in the brain that contain cerebral fluid that "bathes" the central nervous system) and puckered, discolored white matter. Its symptoms are similar to MID's and almost always appears in those with hypertension. In fact, before the advent of the CT scan, it was very difficult to distinguish Binswanger's disease from MID prior to a postmortem. While MID, however, manifests for the most part in those from sixty to seventy-five years of age, Binswanger's disease manifests in those from fifty to seventy.

Inflammatory diseases of the blood vessels. The most common of these is systemic lupus erythematosus (SLE), an autoimmune disorder in which the body's defense system "turns" against itself. It affects many more women than men and can be difficult to diagnose.

Disorders of cerebral blood flow. In extracranial occlusive disease, arteries leading to the brain (the carotid arteries, as well as some vertebral arteries) undergo *stenosis*, a narrowing or tightening. While the resulting decrease in blood flow generally results in a stroke, in an acute setting, it sometimes presents itself as delirium.

Extracranial occlusive disease is probably the closest we come to a dementia produced by a phrase no longer used in discussing the brain, "hardening of the arteries." Clinical features a doctor would discover are bruits (the French word for "noise," a *bruit* is an abnormal sound that would be heard with a stethoscope) and inequality of blood pressure in the upper limbs.

Other disorders that affect cerebral blood flow are aortic arch syndrome, extasia of the basilar artery, arteriovenus malformations, and multiple small-vessel occlusions.

A word about cerebral insufficiency. While the medical profession isn't entirely satisfied with this term, it helps distinguish a condition short of dementia in which cerebral function is impaired—*perhaps reversibly so*.

Symptoms in someone with cerebral insufficiency are usually subtle, and can often be mistaken for those of mild depression. Concentration is impaired, and new tasks are daunting. At times, even familiar tasks just seem to be too much trouble to undertake; the patient frequently becomes impatient and irritable. (You can see why this condition looks so much like mild depression!) Keep in mind however, that someone can have both a medical cause for dementia and depression.

It's believed that these symptoms are somehow connected with a reduced blood flow since they often occur in those who have had heart attacks, clearing up weeks, or possibly months, later. Cardiac arrhythmias (irregular heartbeats) can also cause this syndrome.

As you can see, it indeed isn't always Alzheimer's. Just as reading about the experiences of families that had a member diagnosed as having probable Alzheimer's can help you recognize and begin to deal with that situation, so, too, can reading about people whose symptoms had another cause.

JONATHAN'S STORY: MEDICATION-INDUCED DEMENTIA

Jonathan was a seventy-two-year-old retired engineer whose family had noticed a slow onset of memory difficulties, problems in finding the right word, and that the pace of his walking, once brisk and confident, had slowed considerably.

Concerned, they consulted a neurologist. When the neurologist took Jonathan's history, information about his health was revealed that gave the doctor vital clues to his present condition.

Twenty years before, Jonathan had had a heart attack. While in the coronary care unit, he became very agitated. He was placed on a high dose of Valium, a common antianxiety drug, and discharged on the same dose, along with cardiac medications. These medications were continued by his internist and by two other doctors when Jonathan was transferred to new locations after job promotions.

Jonathan had started taking these medications regularly years before he showed any symptoms of dementia. He went through the full diagnostic process, and no other possible cause of dementia emerged. The neurologist *slowly* tapered Jonathan off the Valium over time, and the symptoms that had led his family to the doctor disappeared. Jonathan's memory difficulties disappeared for the most part, as did his problem in finding the right word. Finally, energy returned to his step. The cumulative effect of years of medication had, indeed, been the cause of his symptoms; fortunately for him, his family sought diagnosis, and both his life and theirs improved.

Jonathan's story underlines these points:

- It can take years for medication-induced dementia to appear. Bring a list of all medications to the doctor, as well as the pill bottles themselves. Tell the doctor how long the medications have been taken and the doses.
- Medical history offers the doctor vital clues to the possible causes of dementia. You may not have connected cardiac problems or medications to dementia symptoms, but the right doctor will. In Chapter Six you'll see how to prepare a patient history *before* you go to the doctor.

AGATHA'S STORY: A MIXED DEMENTIA

Agatha, a retired sixty-eight-year-old teacher, became apathetic and started to withdraw socially, showing a lack of interest and energy. Both her ability to concentrate and her appetite decreased, and she developed insomnia. Along with these symptoms, she also developed memory problems and appeared confused at times. Her husband, noting these changes, took her to the family doctor, who discovered that Agatha had high blood pressure; he suspected that she might be showing the first symptoms of vascular dementia. He decided to start her on medication to lower her blood pressure immediately, since that is such a dangerous condition.

He was concerned, however, that vascular dementia might not, indeed, be the sole culprit. An internist, he knew enough about memory disorders to realize that he could not conduct a complete diagnosis. He referred Agatha to a nearby psychiatrist who had a special interest in memory disorders, and to whom he had previously referred patients, who had been pleased by the thoroughness of the psychiatrist's approach.

On taking Agatha's history, the psychiatrist learned that she had experienced three prior depressions (at ages eighteen, thirty, and forty-five). They had been characterized by a flat and apathetic mood, but without any memory problems or confusion. He also discovered that Agatha's father had had a history of depression, as had an aunt, her father's sister.

The psychiatrist made a diagnosis of major depression. The dementia that results from such a depression is referred to as pseudodementia.

The psychiatrist started Agatha on antidepressants and a brief course of psychotherapy to identify the stresses in her life that preceded this most recent onset of depression. They included her retirement from a career to which she had been devoted, and her two grown children having to move quite a distance away around the same time, her son taking the beloved only grandchild with him.

The psychiatrist also knew that the internist had found that Agatha had high blood pressure. He was not surprised when an MRI revealed some infarctions, or small strokes. Consequently, while a number of her symptoms lifted after a few months, some, notably her memory problems, did not entirely disappear. In addition to major depression, she was diagnosed as being in an early stage of vascular dementia. She was directed to continue her blood pressure medication, to eat more sensibly, and to start exercising. He also had her take ginkgo biloba, an herb shown to help some people who have vascular dementia. Her condition seemed to stabilize, her memory problems not becoming worse.

Agatha's story underlines this point:

• A good doctor is one who knows his limitations. While Agatha's internist discovered she had high blood pressure and knew that this condition could be responsible for her symptoms, he referred her to someone with much more experience and skill in this area, since he was aware that something else could be causing some, or all, of her symptoms.

MRS. JANEWAY'S STORY:
CATCHING A MISDIAGNOSIS

In his memoir, *When Air Hits Your Brain,* neurosurgeon Frank Vertosick, Jr., tells a cautionary tale of misdiagnosis and its eventual correction.

Called one day to his hospital's clinic to examine a Mrs. Janeway, Dr. Vertosick found a sixty-seven-year-old former business dynamo in almost a total stupor. She'd been in a nursing home for several years, having been diagnosed with Alzheimer's. She was sent to the clinic when a young aide there noticed a large bump on the back of her head while combing her hair.

In looking at her records, Dr. Vertosick was surprised to see that she'd been diagnosed with Alzheimer's without having had a brain scan. He ordered one, and it revealed a large, benign (noncancerous) tumor called a meningioma, a type easily removed. Now, it was entirely possible that Mrs. Janeway had both the tumor and Alzheimer's. And after speaking to one of her grown daughters, Dr. Vertosick agreed with her that it was fruitless to put such an ill woman through the operation. But the case was on the doctor's mind all night, and, it turned out, on her daughter's. After speaking with her again, Dr. Vertosick operated, removing the tumor. He now sees Mrs. Janeway once a year—when she pays a whirlwind visit to his office, dressed in a stylish business suit.

Mrs. Janeway's story underlines these points:

- All steps of the diagnosis process *must* be taken. You know that people can have a mixed dementia, that discovering one cause before the diagnosis has been completed does not exclude a second cause. Radiologic examinations are a vital part of the diagnosis.

- It pays to be observant and to follow through on hunches. The saving of Mrs. Janeway depended first on the concern of an aide in a nursing home, the person who noticed the bump on her head, and acted on the observation. Further, both the doctor and Mrs. Janeway's daughter decided to proceed only after the hunch that the tumor may be entirely responsible for her condition had been on their minds overnight.

FOUR

FINDING AND WORKING WITH
THE RIGHT DOCTOR FOR YOU

In this chapter you'll read about how to do something that will be invaluable throughout your loved one's illness. It's gathering information. The first step of course, is to find sources of good information. When it comes to Alzheimer's and other dementias, there is an outstanding source of information—and it's only a phone call away.

THE PHONE CALL THAT GETS YOU STARTED

To contact this tremendous resource, all you have to do is phone 1-800-272-3900, the toll-free national number of an invaluable organization, the Alzheimer's Disease and Related Disorders Association (ADRDA—also referred to as the Alzheimer's Association).

Note that the association does not specialize in Alzheimer's alone. You can get vital information from the time you begin the quest for a diagnosis, as well as continued support if your loved one's symptoms are caused by something other than Alzheimer's.

The association has over 200 chapters nationwide; when you phone the 800 number listed above, ask for the chapter nearest you or your loved one, and ask to be put on the mailing list for the national association's quarterly newsletter.

All chapters have the same *free* core services. These include:

1. *A helpline*—A phone call will put you in direct contact with a trained volunteer. Many of the helplines operate twenty-four hours a day, which is especially useful if it's difficult for you to make phone calls during the work day.
2. *Education*—Your chapter will offer everything from basic information, to news about the latest breakthroughs, to free legal and financial services. Also available are informative, clearly written brochures on a wide variety of topics pertaining to dementing disorders.
3. *Support groups*—Giving care to a person with dementia is emotionally taxing and, all too often, isolating. Association group members give each other information, support and the knowledge that others know what they're going through.
4. *A quarterly newsletter*—Every three months, you'll receive a newsletter that can only be described as a lifeline. It's free to those who cannot pay, and a donation of $5.00 (or more, if you can afford it) to those who can.

CONTACTING THE ALZHEIMER'S ASSOCIATION

1. Buy a spiral-bound notebook so you can have all the information you'll be writing down in one place. A bright cover will make it easy to find in your home.
2. Buy a large envelope or a bright folder with pockets so you can keep papers you gather in one place.
3. If the patient takes a number of prescription medications, a shoebox (or the type of box you can buy in a stationery store to put photos in) will be useful. Here you can keep the patient's most recent prescription pill bottles to take to your first doctor's appointment (the doctor must know what medications the patient has been taking in recent years). If there aren't enough bottles to call for a box, a bright plastic bag will serve.
4. Take out the notebook. On top of a page, write the association's toll-free number—1-800-272-3900. Phone and ask:
   • For the address and phone number of the nearest local chapter.
   • For the helpline number of that chapter.
   • To be put on the mailing list to receive the newsletter.
5. Phone your local chapter (or the local chapter of the person to be diagnosed, if he/she doesn't reside near you). Ask for:
   • Referrals to physicians in the area and if there are any diagnostic centers nearby (these are

often called "memory disorder centers," and
they are usually near large hospitals).

- Referrals to good adult day centers in the
  area.
- Referrals to good attorneys who specialize in
  elder care issues.

Please note: Many chapters do not officially
recommend doctors, day centers, or attorneys.
However you can speak more informally with
members about these kinds of referrals. More
information about finding doctors and other
professionals follows in this chapter.

WHAT DIAGNOSING AND TREATING MEMORY DISORDERS CALLS FOR IN A DOCTOR

Diagnosing and treating any memory disorder is an
involved and time-consuming process. As shown in
Chapter Six, diagnosis alone requires quite a range of
tests. The medical treatment of Alzheimer's also takes
time and effort, as discussed in Chapter Seven, as well
as keeping up with the ever-growing body of knowledge about the disease. Further, as a chronic and degenerative illness, Alzheimer's affects not just the
health of the patient, but many aspects of the life of
both the patient and the patient's family.

The best treatment calls for a doctor who can guide
the patient and family in dealing with more than just
the medical aspects of the disease. It also demands one
capable of guiding them to resources for coping with

the psychological aspects. This means acknowledging the emotional side of the illness and coping with it through such means as individual and/or family therapy and support groups for caregivers. It also means referring patients and families to resources for coping with the sociological aspects, to such community services as adult day centers.

Too Many Doctors—Even Good Ones— Don't Know How to Help Patients and Families Cope with Alzheimer's

Unfortunately, even many fine physicians think that, once a diagnosis of probable Alzheimer's has been reached, that's it. Knowledge in this area of medicine has grown tremendously in the past few years, so unless doctors specialize in caring for the elderly, or have a strong interest in the disease, they won't be aware of all that is available and won't pursue the range of treatment options available today. Incorrectly assuming that they will not make a difference in the course of the illness or in the patient's quality of life, many do not even prescribe one of the two Alzheimer's-specific drugs, Aricept and Cognex.

And many do not address the family's needs at all.

Can you turn at this time to your primary care physician?

It takes quite a body of knowledge to diagnose Alzheimer's, then to give the best possible treatment for it. To do so requires dealing with a number of other professionals, including but not limited to other doctors, psychologists and social workers. If you are concerned about a loved one's possibly having Alzheimer's, think about your relationship with your primary care physician (or your loved one's with his or her physician). Turn to this doctor if you trust that he or she can get you into the right hands to deal with all the aspects of Alzheimer's, and can, indeed, "quarterback" the diagnostic and treatment team.

DIAGNOSTIC CENTERS: THE TEAM APPROACH UNDER ONE ROOF

Diagnosing Alzheimer's and then addressing all the needs of the patient and family are best served by a team approach. Sometimes that team can be led by a primary care physician, an internist or family doctor, or by a geriatrician, neurologist, or psychiatrist. Frequently, it's best to turn to a diagnostic center, often called a memory disorder clinic or center. These have a full complement of necessary professionals on staff; for instance, it is not uncommon for a doctor, a geriatric nurse, and a social worker to be present when the diagnosis is given to the patient and family. They answer the family's immediate questions, refer them to a range of medical and social services, and can handle future questions.

Diagnostic centers are connected with many suburban hospitals throughout the country and with the major urban teaching and research hospitals affiliated with medical schools. In fact, both suburban centers and individual doctors refer cases that are especially difficult to diagnose to the teaching hospitals.

FINDING THE RIGHT DOCTOR
OR DIAGNOSTIC CENTER: IF YOU'RE IN
A MANAGED CARE PLAN

A number of managed plans no longer require you to go through the primary care physician to reach a specialist. If you are in this type of plan you will want to use the techniques described below to get the names of recommended specialists and/or of memory disorder centers near your loved one.

However, in many managed care plans, such as HMOs, all visits to specialists must be cleared by the primary care physician. And unfortunately, some plans put the pressure of the pocketbook on doctors to discourage their referring patients to specialists. If your plan requires that you go to a "gatekeeper" primary care physician, do so.

If You're Not Happy with Your Primary Care Physician in a Managed Care Plan

You may find yourself unhappy with this physician's handling of the case. He may want to diagnose the patient entirely by himself, for instance, or she may not want to have the full range of diagnostic tests completed, thinking she has identified the source of the patient's symptoms early on in the process.

If you are not satisfied, you have the right to insist on an appropriate referral. If you continue to have difficulties with the primary care physician, you have the right to change primary care physicians within your plan. You may have to be very assertive in seeking the right treatment, but keep in mind how much is at stake. You know that diagnosis is vital, that the best care simply cannot begin until the cause, or causes, of symptoms are identified.

Steps to Take When You're Not Satisfied with Your Doctor

Buy a small notebook and use it to keep detailed notes of your requests and the doctor's response to them; these notes will be valuable in both phone and written contact with your managed care plan.

Honestly assess your own communication skills and assertiveness. If you know, for instance, that these aren't your strong points, a relative or friend who is articulate and assertive should make the phone calls to the plan and/or write to them. Of course, you must provide this person with complete information and try to be present during such calls, though this could be difficult if they must be placed during work hours.

Insurers often respond more favorably to courteous requests than to those that are belligerent from the very beginning. However, if you find your requests refused after a detailed, pleasant, and firm presentation, let the insurer know that you plan to go directly to the state insurance commission and/or your senator and congressional representative with your concerns. Such a statement may in itself result in your requests being met; if not, proceed as you've stated you will.

The emotional and tactical support of people who have "been there" can be invaluable. Contact your local chapter of the Alzheimer's Association if you haven't already. Ask members for help in coping with these difficulties.

GETTING THE NAMES OF RECOMMENDED DOCTORS AND DIAGNOSTIC CENTERS

Whenever you're looking for a doctor to handle a specific situation, ideal recommendations come from people who have themselves recently—and successfully—faced the problem. They know the doctor from the patient's perspective. Further, excellent recommendations come from those in the medical profession as well. The first step below shows you how to contact people who have just coped with memory disorders in loved ones. The others present ways to get recommendations from health care professionals.

A SPECIAL NOTE FOR THOSE WHO LIVE FAR FROM THEIR LOVED ONES: The end of this chapter has information specifically for you. However, most of the below suggestions involve using the telephone, and work for those coping long-distance as well as for those whose loved one lives nearby. Make sure to have the name of the county in which your loved one lives, as well as the town name and zip code, when you place your calls.

SOURCES FOR THE NAMES OF RECOMMENDED DOCTORS

A number of the suggestions below call for using the telephone. Some people are very good at getting information on the phone, and some simply aren't. If you fall into that second group, ask someone with good communication skills to make these calls on your behalf. Write out clearly all the necessary information for the person helping you, since you may not be able to be present when the calls are made (most must be made during working hours).

The Alzheimer's Association

The Alzheimer's Disease and Related Disorders Association (ARDRA) is usually referred to in the world in general, and in this book, as the Alzheimer's Association. If you have not yet phoned the Association's 800 number to get information about contacting the chapter closest to your loved one, do so immediately. (In the opening pages of this chapter, you'll find specific information about contacting the association.)

It is not the stated policy of the association to give out the names of doctors. One purpose of the organization however, is for people to share their experiences and information in coping with memory disorders in loved ones. They are a valuable source of information. Members can give you inside information on their experiences with nearby doctors and/or diagnostic centers. You can request the names and phone numbers of people with whom to speak, or, if possible, attend a meeting at the local chapter and discuss your concerns with people there.

The Hospital Closest to You or Your Loved One

Your closest hospital will usually have at least one professional knowledgeable about memory disorders. Phone the geriatric unit at the hospital and ask about the geriatric services. This could be a free-standing department or run by the Department of Internal Medicine, Family Medicine, Neurology, or Psychiatry. Not only the director of the department will be able to give you information; the person who answers the phone or a nurse in the department could be a good source (see information that follows), as would a "Doctor Finder" service at the hospital.

If the hospital you call has its own memory disorder center, speak with experienced people before you go to that center. Many a time has a person with experience suggested a center other than the one absolutely nearest the patient.

Nurses

Nurses are an invaluable source of information, and some nurses specialize in gerontology. Per the preceding point, contact at the local hospital about geriatric services or a school of nursing in your state. Further, many adult day centers have at least one geriatric nurse on staff; see the following regarding contacting adult day centers.

Adult Day Centers

Due to growing need, many counties in highly populated areas have at least one adult day center. The director of such a center, as well as other staff members, may be able to give you the names of good doctors and/or memory disorder centers in the area. You can even request a meeting with the director or with a nurse on the staff. There are several ways to find these centers:

- Phone the hospital closest to your loved one. If this hospital does not have such a center, someone there should be able to refer you to the nearest one.
- Phone the Eldercare Locator at 1-800-677-1116 be-

tween the hours of 9 A.M. and 8 P.M., eastern standard
time. An information specialist will be able to give
you the phone numbers of government sources, usually on both the county and state levels. Make sure
to have the name of your loved one's town and
county, as well as the zip code, ready.

- Most counties now have a board of social services,
  as well as an office created specifically to address the
  concerns of senior citizens. The Eldercare Locator
  can give you the names and number of such offices
  near your loved one. Or, if you live near your loved
  one, you can check your phone book or phone the
  local directory assistance for listings. If you phone a
  county's general office of social services, as opposed
  to an organization specializing in senior services, ask
  to speak with someone familiar with services for the
  elderly.
- Consult *The National Directory of Adult Day Care
  Centers* via your local library or the local chapter of
  the Alzheimer's Association. If neither of those carries the directory, phone the Benjamin B. Green-Field
  Library of the main office of the Alzheimer's
  Association, which is in Chicago. The number of the
  Green-Field Library is 312-335-5767; the hours are
  8:30 A.M. to 5 P.M., central standard time.

People You Know

Think about the people you know, or those whom
people close to you may know. Is there anyone in your
neighborhood, church, temple, mosque, or any other organizations, who may be familiar with the local medical
community? A current or retired doctor or nurse, or
perhaps a current or former employee of a hospital or

a doctor's office? Such a person may well be able to give you some useful information.

WHAT TO LOOK FOR IN A RECOMMENDED DOCTOR OR DIAGNOSTIC CENTER

Once you have the names of several recommended doctors and/or centers, you'll want to think about the following three points (in the case of memory disorder centers, these questions apply to the doctor there who is coordinating the diagnosis and care of your loved one):

1. Credentials.
2. Orientation toward treatment.
3. Your working relationship with the doctor.

1. Credentials

   First of all, are the doctors you're considering board certified?

   Where did they do their residencies? (This is a more important consideration for clinical skills and knowledge of a specialty than their medical schools.)

   What is the depth of their specific interest and training in dementia?

   What about their academic/medical school and hospital appointments?

   Have they published or lectured in this area?
2. Orientation Toward Treatment

   Some doctors are aggressive in treatment, some conservative, some middle of the road. It's important, however, that your doctor share your approach.

A Possible Area of Contention:
Approaches to Medication

There has been an explosion of information about treating Alzheimer's in just the past few years. And by the time you've finished reading this book, you'll be knowledgeable about it.

You'll have read, for instance, about the two Alzheimer's-specific drugs, both approved by the FDA only in this decade, as well as of the off-label use of drugs approved by the FDA for other conditions to treat Alzheimer's itself. An example of this is treating Alzheimer's patients with estrogen hormone replacement therapy (a use now being studied for FDA approval), while the current approved use is to treat symptoms of menopause. You will also have read about treating the behavioral symptoms of Alzheimer's with drugs developed for other conditions with similar symptoms. Finally, you'll be acquainted with the use of nondrug substances such as antioxidant vitamins and herbs such as gingko biloba in the battle against Alzheimer's. (These treatment options are discussed in Chapter Seven.)

You may very well want a doctor who is aware of the range of treatments available, or who is willing to learn about them, *and* who is willing to treat the disease as aggressively as you deem necessary. Or, you may indeed be more conservative in approach than a particular doctor, and don't feel comfortable with the treatment suggested. Either way, it's best for your loved one when you and the doctor have a similar view of treatment issues.

3. Your working relationship with the doctor
Once you're satisfied with a particular doctor's

credentials and treatment orientation, this final point merits your attention. To get the best care for your loved one, you must have a good working relationship with the doctor. A good working relationship, on your side, means one in which you feel free to raise any concerns or questions you may have, and either the doctor or a member of the office staff addresses them to your satisfaction; it's one in which such questions or concerns are raised appropriately— you don't sit on them for a long time, then explode with rage or another strong emotion when you can hold them in no longer. It also means that *one* member of the family is the contact person with the doctor, that a number of different people don't phone throughout the day for updates.

In short, it means that you and the doctor get along.

One problem in this area, for instance, are doctors who look good "on paper," and people's awe of them. Of course, everyone wants the best for loved ones. Often however, when it comes to doctors, "best" means how they handle our particular situation. A doctor may be well known in his field, may speak all over the country or even the world, and have published frequently. Yet if he's not available to you and to the patient, those achievements start to pale. A doctor may be brusque, possibly hurried, and make you feel inadequate or stupid to be asking questions. Or he or she may be too laid back, may not be showing the interest and expertise in the patient in particular and the field of dementia in general that would result in the best treatment available.

Obviously, a doctor may be unacceptable in a variety of ways relating to communication with you or treatment of the patient and you.

Any problem with a doctor can be a difficult situation for a number of reasons. First of all, whenever there's an on-going illness in a family, tensions run high. Second, doctors are powerful authority figures, and many people don't feel comfortable bringing up their concerns.

In the next chapter, you'll see how to get your family to work together when a member has a memory disorder. Note in particular how you must be organized as a family when dealing with the doctor and the office staff. If you find that you're following the suggestions offered, have requested changes in unacceptable behavior on the part of the doctor and the office staff, and are still feeling dissatisfied, you must find the courage to cope appropriately with your concerns.

If you do not have a good working relationship with a doctor, do not stay with that doctor.

To cope with this situation, look back to the earlier section in this chapter titled, ''Finding the Right Doctor or Diagnostic Center: If You're in a Managed Care Plan.'' You'll find that you can adapt information from the last two parts, ''If You're Not Happy with Your Primary Care Physician in a Managed Care Plan'' and ''Steps to Take When You're Not Satisfied with Your Doctor.''

Remember, the well being of your loved one is at stake. Go back to the list of names you compiled in your original search for a doctor, and contact a new one. There's a good chance you'll be astonished, and vastly relieved, by the result of your actions.

WHEN THE PATIENT LIVES FAR AWAY, PART ONE—COPING ON YOUR OWN

As noted earlier in this chapter under ''Getting the Names of Recommended Doctors and Diagnostic Centers,'' in a special note to those who live far from their loved ones, many of the sources discussed there are as valuable for those living far from the patient as they are for those who live mere minutes away. The telephone is a great tool for gathering information at any distance.

There comes a time, however, when you—or another member of the family, or a family friend—just has to be there.

There are two keys to long-distance coping:

1. Gathering information and making necessary appointments in advance.
2. Coordinating family members' roles and responsibilities.

Your primary concern is diagnosis and your next concern is coping with the steps you must take in the wake of that diagnosis. The date of your trip will be determined to a great extent by the availability of experts near your loved one, especially by the dates of the initial diagnostic work. So, *before you finalize your travel plans, you need*:

1. An appointment with a recommended physician or memory disorder center in your loved one's area.
2. To have contacted the local government organization or social services agency that handles cases in your loved one's locale to get information in advance on

what's available. You should also set up an appointment with someone there to get information in person.

3. The name and phone number of at least one recommended adult day center near your loved one; it's a good idea to schedule a meeting with the appropriate person there before you leave home.

4. Names and phone numbers of recommended attorneys who specialize in elder care issues. Find out the fee for an initial appointment; you may well wish to have such an appointment on this trip.

The most direct ways to accomplish the above? Have ready the name of your loved one's state, county, town and zip code. Phone the toll-free national number of the Alzheimer's Association—1-800-272-3900—as discussed in the opening of this chapter. Someone there will be able to give you the number of the chapter closest to your loved one. Members of that chapter should be an excellent source of information for the above. You can also phone the toll-free number of the Eldercare Locator—1-800-677-1116—between 9 A.M. and 8 P.M. eastern standard time. This source will give you names and phone numbers of state and local government organizations that serve the elder population as well as names and phone numbers of adult day centers.

WHEN YOU NEED MORE THAN INFORMATION: HANDLING A PATIENT'S (AND FAMILY'S) RESISTANCE

Perhaps one of the factors that's been getting in the way of your helping someone with a memory disorder is the would-be patient's resistance to even an initial visit to the doctor. If that's the case, you'll need one more thing before you depart—a strategy to get your loved one to cooperate. Further, if other family members are also showing resistance, you'll need to cope with them. You will read in detail about the issue of patient and family resistance in the next chapter, "Handling Difficulties with the Patient and/or Other Family Members."

The below story however, tells how a grown son, long concerned about his father's growing impairment but frustrated in any attempt to cope effectively with it, learned specific steps to take to get his father diagnosed and to get both his parents' future on the right track.

BOB'S STORY: COPING LONG DISTANCE WITH A RESISTANT PATIENT AND FAMILY

By the time they were all in their forties, Bob Harrison and his sisters, Gail and Kate, each lived several hours from their elderly parents—Bob was in Boston, Gail in California, Kate in Florida, and their parents, Peter and Elizabeth, outside Chicago. Since Bob was in Chicago every three months or so on business, he saw his parents much more frequently than his sisters did. After three visits spaced over ten months, Bob had to acknowledge that something was wrong with his father. He was obviously experiencing real problems with memory loss.

Yet when Bob tried to discuss his concerns with Gail and Kate they did not take him seriously, claiming that of course their father wasn't going to be as sharp as he'd been before—he was seventy-three, after all—but that didn't mean he was sick. And Bob knew that speaking with his mother about his concerns would be fruitless. His father had always handled any difficult issue within the family, priding himself on protecting his wife. Bob knew he'd have to handle things as best he could.

Without knowing what doctor to go to and without a strategy for getting his father to go even if he knew of one, Bob just became more and more frustrated each time he visited his parents. And now he was starting to get concerned about his mother. Though Elizabeth never complained openly, Bob could tell what a strain it was for her to handle his father, who had to have someone with him every minute of the day and who seemed to be acting more and more like a very big child.

One day at work Bob was lucky enough to overhear a woman talking about her mother, who was in an adult day center. That woman gave him the toll-free number of the Alzheimer's Association. Bob phoned and was put in touch with the chapter nearest Peter and Elizabeth. Members told him about a good memory disorder center less than an hour from his parents' house. He called and made an appointment for his father that coincided with his next business trip. Equally important, they gave him a strategy to get Peter to go to the center. Bob should say that he was concerned about his parents' health as well as his own, and tell them that he had scheduled general check-ups for all of them.

The evening before the appointment he privately told his mother what he was doing. To his surprise, she expressed relief (which only shows you that frequently, people are more aware of things than we give them credit for, even if it seems that they are not). The next day, Elizabeth drove while Bob rode with his father in the back seat. Bob knew his father well and was especially aware of his father's pride in taking care of his wife and of his need to protect her. He appealed to those instincts in his father, telling him that he had been worried about his health for a bit but that he was especially concerned about the effect his father's ill health could have on Elizabeth. The only possible thing to do was have a doctor assess the problem. Bob's knowledge of his father was accurate; Peter showed absolutely no resistance and in fact also seemed relieved at being attended to, especially by the pleasant but obviously competent doctor who ran the center.

When Peter's diagnosis of probable Alzheimer's was finalized after a variety of tests (described in Chapter Six), he was put on the drug Aricept by a physician recommended by the center. He showed improvement within about six weeks and shortly thereafter his dosage was increased, resulting in further improvement. At this point, the physician introduced high doses of Vitamin E; he planned to introduce further treatments step by step, both to see which ones made a difference, and also to watch out for any side effects.

Before he had to return to Boston, Bob met with the geriatric nurse who directed a nearby adult day center. It had been recommended by a number of people he'd met through the local Alzheimer's Association, as well as by several people at the diagnostic center. To Bob's relief, his father would be able to go to the center two days a week and possibly more often in a few months. And since their parents did not qualify for government assistance in paying for those two days, Bob's sister Gail, the most financially successful of the three siblings, offered to meet this expense. Her attitude had been changed by her mother, who now discussed Peter's declining state with her daughters on the phone.

Like their father Gail was very concerned about taking care of Elizabeth. As a further extension of this concern, Gail made time in a demanding business schedule to fly out two weeks after Bob had had to get back to Boston to take her mother to an attorney to make arrangements for her future. Bob and Kate acknowledged that Gail was the best suited of the three of them to handle this kind of meeting and to take care of their parents' financial and legal concerns.

Kate, the youngest sibling but the only one with children, made plans to come out for a month as soon as her sons were on summer vacation. Both Peter and Elizabeth had always greatly enjoyed seeing their two grandchildren, but Kate had put off such trips several times in the past. Her father's illness made her aware that she wouldn't have her parents forever and she would now take every opportunity for her and the boys to see them. Since her family finances were tight, the expense of this trip was also met by Gail.

Within a few months of Bob's taking Peter to the doctor, everyone was better off.

Bob's story underlines these points:

* In the face of patient and family resistance, one person's taking action can be vital; Bob's early efforts had a domino effect on his family, breaking through their denial.
* Successful early actions depend on gathering information and planning in advance; only after Bob learned how to do this was he able to get his father diagnosed.

- If there's resistance to seeking help, come up with a strategy in advance.
- This is a team effort; all do not have to (and indeed cannot) contribute in the same way. Devise a workable division of tasks.
- As always, it's diagnosis that leads to a bettering of the patient's situation, and the spouse's. Peter's medical treatment, his placement in a good adult day center a few days a week, Elizabeth's improvement due to respite, and all the siblings getting a stronger awareness of family, that they had to enjoy their family now—none of these would have happened without a diagnosis.

WHEN THE PATIENT LIVES FAR AWAY, PART TWO—HIRING A PROFESSIONAL

In Part One of this section, you read about a grown son who managed to get his father diagnosed and who then got his two sisters to help out with post-diagnosis issues. However, if you don't have any other family members, or if you do, but none of them can or will help—and if you have the funds—you can turn to a professional geriatric care manager. For instance if Gail, the very successful businesswoman in the anecdote above, had had no siblings, this would have been a good course of action for her to investigate.

With graduate training in the field of human services (gerontology, nursing, social work, or psychology), these care managers can be invaluable. In fact, they are not solely a choice for those living far from the patient, but they can also be of help to those who live nearby. Their services include:

- Assessment
- Arrangements for home care
- Care management and long-term monitoring
- Help with nursing home placement
- Counseling
- Crisis intervention
- Access to entitlements and services
- Financial management

HOW TO LOCATE A PROFESSIONAL CARE MANAGER

Using the contacts mentioned earlier in this chapter in "Sources for the Names of Recommended Doctors," network with people who have hired such care managers to see if you can get some recommendations. You can also contact:

The National Association of Professional Geriatric Care Managers
655 North Alvernon Way, Suite 108
Tucson, AZ 85711
(602) 881-8008

FIVE

HANDLING DIFFICULTIES WITH THE PATIENT AND/OR OTHER FAMILY MEMBERS

You've picked up this book because you've been aware of certain changes in a loved one, changes that tell you that something fairly serious is wrong. You may have been thinking about these changes for a while, even for a year or more. You may even have been hoping that you haven't really been seeing what you know, deep down, you've been seeing.

Your reading this book shows that you're ready to face reality. However, the would-be patient, and possibly other family members, may not yet be at that stage.

RESISTANCE TO GOING TO THE DOCTOR— A COMMON REACTION

There's a good chance that the symptoms that concern you aren't the only things you have to cope with right now. In fact, you may have already tried to get

the person you're worried about to see a doctor, and
have met a lot of resistance.

This situation is more common than you might think.
Refusing to acknowledge memory impairment is a big
part of denying aging itself. It's also difficult to accept
changing roles in the family. For instance, a parent who
has spent a lifetime taking care of others often does not
want to acknowledge needing help—especially help
from a grown child. An affected spouse may be the
person who used to force you to go to the doctor, or
could be someone who hasn't been to a doctor since
his days in the army—decades ago.

AND RESISTANCE DOESN'T COME JUST FROM THE WOULD-BE PATIENT

It's also possible that the would-be patient is not the
only one getting in the way of dealing with the problems you've noticed. If it's your spouse who concerns
you, one (or more) of your grown children may swear,
"Nothing's wrong with Dad!" Or it may be one of your
spouse's siblings, perhaps the brother who never
thought you were good enough for his baby sister, and
wasn't he right—here you are, claiming she has some
kind of problem and trying to railroad her off.

You may be trying to cope with a parent's symptoms,
only to find that years of long simmering, never resolved sibling rivalry has come to the surface. "You
never got along with Mom," is an accusation you may
hear from a favored son regarding anything *his* mother
does that you raise any questions about. Or, you may
be hit with, "There's nothing wrong with Dad—we had
a great conversation last night"—when, if brother had

stayed over more than one evening, he would have heard that same "great conversation" several times.

DENIAL—A COPING MECHANISM THAT GETS IN THE WAY OF COPING

People who deny reality in this way aren't being malicious, trying to get back at you after years of resentments. They are caught up in *denial*, the phenomenon discussed on page 11 of Chapter One, under the heading "Noting Symptoms in a Loved One—Not as Easy as it Might Seem."

Remember, denial is an *unconscious* defense mechanism; people in denial are not aware that they are denying the existence of facts—they simply are not yet able to accept those facts on a conscious level.

COPING WITH DIFFICULT FAMILY MEMBERS

Yes, there are ways of approaching this type of resistance, of breaking through the blocks that are getting in the way of your taking care of a loved one. They can be divided into three factors.

The Three Factors That Can Help You Get a Dementia Patient Evaluated

They are discussed here briefly; you'll read about them in greater detail below.

1. *Consensus (agreement) with the spouse and/or within the family*. No matter how difficult it can be

to deal with certain people in your family, keep in mind that a feeling of ambiguity or even of conflict in family members increases the resistance and ambivalence in a patient with a potentially serious illness. Getting the major players to cooperate is an important first step in having the patient diagnosed and treated. Yet where do you start when trying to get all these (doubtless) difficult people known as your family to cooperate? Here's where the next factor comes into play.

2. *The personality types of both the patient and of family members*. Health care professionals know that, to motivate people, it helps to take their basic personality types into account. Doing so can help you decide how best to get people to work together productively.

3. *The particular symptoms of an individual's dementia*. Not everyone's dementia is the same. Some people seem primarily confused, some depressed, others anxious, passive or withdrawn. These are the dominant symptoms of dementia; they cause the affected person to react better to certain approaches than to others.

A SPECIAL WORD FOR THOSE COPING WITHOUT FAMILY

You may be in a time of life when you don't have close relatives, when, indeed, the person with whom you're closest in the world—most likely your spouse, or your sole surviving parent, or a much loved sibling—is undergoing the difficulties that led you to this book.

Please know that we're aware that your experience is especially difficult, and our thoughts are with you. You're going to have to be stronger and more resourceful than most who are reading this book. It is you who will have to take the bull by the horns yourself and get moving on diagnosis and follow through.

All those touched by this disease will benefit from involvement with their local chapter of the Alzheimer's Association, as well as other contacts they may have from work (or from their working years), and from religious and social organizations. You will find these resources especially valuable. Further, your county or state may well have services that will help you in this toughest of times. For some guidance in reaching the right offices, contact the Alzheimer's Association and the Eldercare Locator (both have 800 numbers listed in Chapter Eight).

Don't try to soldier on alone. You'll be better able to take care of your loved one if you are at your best. For instance, even a few hours of respite from caregiving can refresh and strengthen you in ways hard to imagine until you actually experience them. You also may consider brief therapy with a specific focus on the unique stresses of dealing with a loved one suffering a memory disorder. A psychiatrist, psychologist, MSW or credentialed counselor would be the right kind of expert. Get referrals from people you've met through the resources mentioned above, those who have recently gone through this experience.

PERSONALITY TYPE: A MAJOR GUIDE TO DEALING WITH OTHERS

Personality is the sum of a person's style of thinking, feeling and behaving. Personality *traits*, qualities or features, are the aspects that make up personality, sometimes referred to as "character." These traits are so much a part of someone that we eventually take them for granted, often not thinking about them consciously.

In fact, these traits are such an intrinsic part of people that we can get to the point where we often take note of people's personalities only when they show traits we *don't* associate with them—when they act "out of character." Dad may normally be the most generous person in the family—so you're startled when he hoards the one box of Godiva chocolate the family got during the holidays, sharing only lesser brands with others. Uncle Bob may, on the other hand, be known as unaccommodating, somewhat selfish, even grouchy. The absence of these traits stands out when he's exceptionally nice to the attractive blonde your brother is dating.

You can use these more unusual behaviors—the ones you tend to notice—to help you hone in on a person's dominant style, on his/her personality type. Think about the sort of behaviors, reactions, etc., that have struck you as being out of character for someone; thinking of their opposites will probably lead you to the person's dominant, more usual style.

TWO POINTS TO KEEP IN MIND CONCERNING PERSONALITY TYPES

1. A number of *types* are discussed below; each person is different, and may have components of several

personality types. In addition, an individual may have traits to greater or lesser degrees. For instance, wanting to be needed and important, to be the center of attention—major traits of Type five—can be expressed subtly, in a quietly commanding way by a powerful but restrained executive, or it can be expressed flagrantly, in a domineering (all right, obnoxious) way by a small business owner who does not have to conform to corporate protocol. The degree to which they express shared traits is a major point in determining the kind of setting in which different people function best.

2. People with Alzheimer's may exhibit a more extreme form of their basic type than before their illness. For instance, someone who has tended to be anxious and needy may show an exaggerated degree of those traits and become clinging. Someone who did not readily trust others may become suspicious to the point of paranoia. People may, on the other hand, show a muted version of their type.

Further, keep in mind that you may have noticed personality changes, traits you've never seen before, including hostility and agitation, and passiveness in the person you're concerned about. You'll read more about this later in this chapter.

SOME BASIC PERSONALITY TYPES AND HOW TO HELP THEM OVERCOME THEIR RESISTANCE TO SEEKING MEDICAL ATTENTION OR TREATMENT

Here you'll see several types described, along with the kind of approach most effective with that type.

You'll see how families can best present health-related issues, such as going to the doctor or to a day center, once they've noticed the sort of symptoms discussed in Chapter One.

Type One

Generally easygoing and pleasant; not overly needy nor overly demanding.

Approach by family members—You're fortunate; people of this type respond well to polite *statements* such as: "Please get ready; we have to leave for a doctor's appointment in about half an hour."

However, be aware that these people may respond very politely, *but in the negative*, to *requests*, which can bring out resistance in them. Don't say, "This is a nice adult center. Would you like to come here while I'm at work?" You'll likely get a direct, polite, "No," in response. If the person simply can't be left alone while you're out of the house, don't pretend that there's a choice. It's much more effective for you to make a statement, such as, "I'm so glad that this center is run by good people, and that everyone here seems so nice. Since it's not safe for you to be alone, I'm relieved we've found such a good place for you to be during the day."

Type Two

Tends to be somewhat anxious and needy; can be fearful in situations that would not inspire fear in most people.

Approach by family members—People of this type respond best when others emphasize that they are doing something *for* the person. Family members might say, for instance, that they have set up an appointment with a highly recommended doctor because they want to take care of the patient and make sure he/she gets the best treatment.

Any demands you must make of people of this personality type should be gentle and firm, but not critical; critical demands will most likely lead to tears and to increased anxiety and fear. Instead of saying, "You must get dressed now since we have to leave for the doctor's office in half an hour," try something along the lines of, "I stayed up extra late last night to make sure these clothes were ready for you for your appointment today; I know how much you like this outfit. I'll help you get dressed. Bob will pick us up; he took the day off because he wanted to be able to drive you."

Type Three

Tends to be a bit unbending, even rigid. Has rather strict rules and expectations. Believes that the letter, not the spirit, of the law is to followed—by everyone, no matter what the circumstances. Is very annoyed by what he/she perceives as irresponsible behavior.

Approach by family members—People of this type respond well when others point out that certain actions (such as taking care of one's health and going to the doctor) constitute doing the right thing. You could say, for instance, that responsible people go for regular medical checkups, and that you don't understand why some people don't follow this basic health rule. You could even point out that it's that kind of irresponsible behavior that drives up everyone's insurance premiums, since people who postpone doctor's appointments don't

have their health problems treated until they're at a
more serious—and costly—stage.

Type Four

Tends to be dramatic and emotional. The stereotypic
actor's personality, larger than life.

Approach by family members—People of this type
respond well to flattery; family members should emphasize what a wonderful thing the person is doing. For
instance, you might say, "It's so great that you'll be
going to the center while Karen's at the office. She's
been worried about your being alone, and it's wonderful
of you to ease her fears. And your being there is going
to be so good for everyone who goes—you're so upbeat
that you'll make all of them feel better."

Type Five

Similar to type four, but with a different emphasis;
Type four responds to being seen as doing wonderful
things; Type five is more self-centered, and wants to be
acknowledged as the most important person in every
setting.

Approach by family members—Since it's vital for
people of this type to feel important, it works best for
family members to emphasize that *they* need the patient's help. An effective statement would be, "We really need your help. We're concerned about a few
things, and you're the only person who can get things
resolved. We've set up a doctor's appointment, and we
need you to go."

It will help if you underline what a top doctor you're

going to see, how hard it was to get an appointment, that this doctor doesn't make time for just anyone, etc.

Type Six

Has trouble trusting others, and is often suspicious of their motivations. Feels much more secure in a situation he/she controls.

Approach by family members—You will find it most effective to make any requests or suggestions in a matter of fact, almost impersonal way, and to phrase them in a way that makes the person think that he/she is in charge and is not taking someone else's advice. For instance, it would be more effective for you to say, "This is what you may consider doing based on the following medical information," than to say, "Mom and I are really concerned about you and want you to go see the doctor."

Do not make demands of people of this personality type, but give a lot of thought to the statements you will make to them, since you want them to conclude that it's best to do what you know is necessary. Again, these people must always think that they are making the decisions, since feeling in control is so vital.

Type Seven

Somewhat withdrawn, could even be seen as a bit eccentric.

Approach by family members—People of this type feel most secure when things are done quietly and privately. For instance, if you've spoken with a number of sources to get names of doctors who are very good at diagnosing memory disorders, don't reveal the scope of your search to the patient, who would not be comfortable knowing that lots of people were contacted regarding his problem.

Emphasize that diagnosis will be handled in a safe, private way.

Type Eight

Very different from Type three, to whom it's important to follow rules, this type frequently disregards them without a second thought.

Approach by family members—People of this type respond best when it's emphasized that any action to be taken would benefit them, rather than, say, any other members of the family, since they don't have a strong sense of responsibility or obligation to others. To get this type of person to go to the first doctor's appointment, you should say, "This may make *you* feel better."

Type Nine

Wants everything to go pleasantly and smoothly (even if the outcome isn't satisfactory!), cannot stand confrontation and retreats from potentially unpleasant situations.

Approach by family members—It's best for the family to emphasize that the doctor's appointment will be quick, and then it will be over. In terms of something like going to an adult day center (which obviously won't be over quickly, since it lasts several hours a day and since the person will attend as many as five days a week), you should emphasize how pleasant the center is.

You can also underscore how both the doctor's appointment and going to a day center will lead to other pleasant things, by planning activities that the person likes (such as quiet walks in a park, or trips to a favorite shop or mall, going out for ice cream, etc.), promising to take the person out on the activity, and *following through*. You can say, "And after the doctor's appointment, let's drive over to that mall you like—you know, the one we don't go to that often." This gives people of this type something pleasant to look forward to, and can help them cope with their desire to avoid what they perceive as potentially unpleasant. (Yes, it's a bribe, but a constructive one, made to help you provide for their health and safety. And remember, no matter what is causing their symptoms, these people are older and you might not otherwise be spending so much time with them. You'll be spared the regret felt by so many people who have wished they'd spent more time with older relatives while it was still possible.)

HOW MEMORY DISORDERS AFFECT PERSONALITY TYPE

As noted earlier, personality traits can be expressed more strongly or more weakly as a result of a memory disorder. People can also regress emotionally, and you will find them using more primitive or immature patterns of relating and behaving.

This regression can be good or bad in terms of your getting people to act in their own self-interest. An independent person may regress to acting like an obedient child. Someone else, on the other hand, may regress to the behavior of a defiant child, and oppose whatever you suggest merely for the sake of opposing it.

At times, you may see both types of regression in the same individual. For instance, someone who is most often obedient will show brief spells of obstinance and rebellion. These fluctuations are often tied to time of day. Alzheimer's patients are frequently agitated very early in the morning—at, say, five a.m.—rising hours before they used to. They will then calm down for most of the day, becoming agitated again near the end of the afternoon. This pattern is known as sun-downing.

AN IMPORTANT NOTE ABOUT SCHEDULING APPOINTMENTS WITH DOCTORS, ATTORNEYS WHO SPECIALIZE IN ELDER LAW, ETC.: ALZHEIMER'S PATIENTS ARE FREQUENTLY AT THEIR BEST FROM SEVEN OR EIGHT A.M. THROUGH THE MORNING. THEREFORE, SCHEDULE ALL MAJOR APPOINTMENTS AS EARLY IN THE MORNING AS POSSIBLE.

An Individual's Particular Symptoms of Dementia: Taking Them into Account When You're Trying to Overcome Their Resistance to Seeking Treatment

As noted earlier, not everyone experiences dementia in the same way. One person's dominant symptom may be confusion, another's memory loss, yet another's anxiety. Different symptoms call for different types of communication. The following are symptoms of dementia that can be dominant in an individual, as well as the type of communication most effective with that symptom.

Dominant symptom	The most effective way to communicate
confused	is brief and clear
memory impairment	is brief, clear and repetitive
paranoid	is direct and without secrecy
depressed	is to take control and ignore helplessness
anxious	is to be calm and reassuring

ORGANIZING YOUR FAMILY TO FACILIATE THE DIAGNOSTIC PROCESS

Factors in addition to individual personality type affect a family's dealing successfuly with both the patient and the medical system.

Answering these questions will give you valuable information about how best to proceed:

1. Are there unresolved sibling issues in your family?
2. What about birth order? Will the oldest take charge, will younger ones be passive or competitive?
3. What about feelings toward authority, in this case personified by the doctor? First borns, for instance, are often noted for heeding authority—after all, as first borns, they are often perceived as authorities within the sibling group, while second borns are much less hesitant to challenge authority. These

characteristics can help determine who is willing to assert him/herself and advocate for the patient.

HOW YOUR FAMILY CAN BEST DEAL WITH DOCTORS AND THEIR STAFFS

You've been reading a lot about your family and their perspective on the difficult process of diagnosing someone with a memory disorder. It's useful to keep in mind the point of view of someone vital to the situation, the doctor.

Diagnosing memory disorders is time consuming, involving a lot of interviews with the patient and family, many medical tests, and coordinating the work of a number of medical professionals. To tell the truth, it's considerable work for which doctors will be receving less than their usual fee, since the vast majority of people in need of this diagnosis will be on Medicare. (Medicare fees are set by the government and are usually much lower than the fee-for-service cost or even the managed care fee.)

The doctor's work will be made much easier if he or she speaks only to one designated family member, instead of having to field calls throughout the day from a number of people in the patient's family.

ASSIGNING SPECIFIC TASKS TO FAMILY MEMBERS

Who is best suited to be the contact person with the doctor's office? This should be someone:

- With a good phone manner.
- Who is accessible during the work day (and/or has a reliable answering machine).
- Who will write things down and communicate them to the rest of the family.

Your particular family situation will determine which tasks are to be assigned. They can include:

1. Family's designated phone contact with doctor/doctor's staff.
2. Person(s) who takes patient to the doctor's office and/or other test locations.
3. Patient's main day-to-day caregiver (often a spouse or a grown child living in or near the family home).
4. Those who relieve the main caregiver.

It's good to set up a schedule for this. For instance, if Bill usually stays with Mother Sunday afternoons, but suddenly finds he can have tickets for a ball game he'd like to see, it's up to him to arrange a change with someone else as soon as possible. He can then somehow help that person with his/her task in exchange.

If you're the person switching with Bill on this occasion, don't keep bringing it up and holding it over his head. Your family is in a difficult situation, and tempers can flare. Keep in mind that you're working together to cope with a family crisis.

Flexibility and creativity in your approach are key. If some family members can't give time on a regular basis, for whatever reason—overburdened with young children, working a full-time job while working part-

time on a degree, simply living too far away—perhaps
they can give something else. This could be money, be
it to enable a distant sibling to fly in, or for care at an
adult day center, or maybe it could be a special, concentrated weekend of respite for the main caregiver or
others who caregive on a regular basis—someone who
lives far away (and whose finances allow) could fly in,
even if just for a weekend, and be the main caregiver
for that weekend, giving others the weekend off. A bo-
nus for this person is the chance to spend time with
someone in the latter years of life, an opportunity that
will eventually be lost.

A COMMON, UNUSUALLY SUCCESSFUL TECHNIQUE FOR GETTING A RESISTANT PERSON TO THE DOCTOR

If you've found after trying the approaches mentioned above that you still can't get your loved one to
the doctor, you can try this one, which a number of
people have found useful:

Get a few family members together—say, one or two
grown children, and the spouse of the affected person—
and say that it's about time that you all went for general
check-ups, to have your blood pressure taken, etc. Medical professionals report that, when this approach is
used, people who would refuse to leave the house for
a doctor's appointment are usually very cooperative.

They may become compliant once at the doctor's because they're putting on their ''company manners''—
resist as they might when alone with family members,
they wouldn't do so in front of strangers, especially
such authority figures as doctors, whose ritualized,

white-coated work attire, private vocabulary and hierarchical way of being addressed serve a valuable function in this kind of situation.

However, an important part of their cooperation at this stage may indeed be a sense of relief that a problem that's hard to even acknowledge among family and friends, let alone talk about or cope with, is finally starting to be taken care of. And now the concerned parties are highly trained professionals who have no personal agenda and no emotional involvement in the complex web of family relationships.

WHEN YOU'RE AT YOUR WIT'S END— WHAT TO DO WHEN THEY ABSOLUTELY REFUSE TO GET HELP

Sometimes, however, not even this approach works, and concerned relatives can feel desperate, that there's absolutely no hope. They don't want Mom to burn down her condo and possibly her neighbors' (she's already had a few fires in her kitchen), or Dad to freeze during his 4 a.m. wanderings through the neighborhood, or Uncle Mike to kill himself and maybe even others in the car he insists on continuing to drive—but they don't know what to do.

These people's status is life-threatening but they simply won't get help. If you look back at the personality types discussed earlier in this chapter, you'll see that many of these people are now showing very extreme manifestations of the traits described, to the point that they have become truly dysfunctional. You know in your heart of hearts that, if they continue in this way, they are posing grave danger to themselves, and even to others.

This is when you have to resort to the solution left to you—having your loved one committed.

HAVING SOMEONE COMMITTED—A REGULATED LEGAL PROCESS, NOT A BANISHMENT TO AN ASYLUM

You may be shrieking right now—that's not something anyone in your family would ever do. After all, you love Mom, Dad or Uncle Mike. Yet we're talking about someone with an illness that has affected his judgment, his very ability to take care of himself in this world. Is leaving someone in that state, in a situation where he faces injury or even death, an expression of love?

Nowadays, commitment is *not* the process we recall from old movies and soap operas, in which vindictive, money-hungry relatives bribe a doctor to consign someone indefinitely to a snake pit. While commitment is, of course, strongly influenced by a physician's assessment—and, usually, the opinion of *two* physicians is needed—it is a *legal* decision.

COMMITMENT REQUIRES THE APPROVAL OF A JUDGE AND, IN MOST STATES, A SECOND MEDICAL ASSESSMENT AND A SECOND LEGAL REVIEW SEVENTY-TWO HOURS AFTER THE INITIAL COMMITMENT. AT THE POINT OF COMMITMENT, THE PATIENT IS ALWAYS ASKED IF HE IS WILLING TO GO VOLUNTARILY INTO A HOSPITAL. MORE OFTEN THAN NOT THEY DO

SO, DISPENSING WITH THE NEED FOR THE IN-
VOLUNTARY COMMITMENT PROCESS.

What Commitment Entails

While the laws regarding commitment vary somewhat from state to state, in general the process works
in this way:

Often, someone—a family member concerned by behavior dangerous to the affected person, or even a member of the general public who has found a wandering,
disoriented person (and this happens, unfortunately,
more frequently than you might think)—calls the local
rescue squad or the police, who take the patient to the
emergency room.

An example of this type of intervention is Phil's
story, told near the end of Chapter One. After receiving
a diagnosis of probable Alzheimer's in a time before
current treatments were available, Phil stayed at home
past the time it was the safest option for him and for
his wife, Janet. One evening, Phil thought Janet was a
thief in their apartment, and he actually became violent.
A neighbor overhearing the fracas called the police, Phil
himself called the police (to have them handle the
"thief"), and their grown daughter, whom Phil had
phoned, realized what was happening and also called
the police. Accustomed to dealing with this kind of situation, the police handled it very well, and took Phil to
a good hospital. Here, after doctors examined him, the
extent of his needs finally became addressed. It was
agreed he could no longer live at home, and he went to
a good nursing home near Janet.

What do physicians look for in assessing such patients? If possible, a physical exam and blood tests are

done in the ER. The legal decision to commit someone depends on the patient's state meeting one of these three criteria:

1. The patient is acutely suicidal (meaning he/she will shortly attempt suicide).
2. The patient is acutely homicidal (meaning that he/she, if left unattended, will shortly attempt to kill someone else).
3. The patient's functioning is so disorganized that, left on his or her own, the patient poses a serious threat to his/her own life.

It is, of course, this third point that pertains to the person suffering from dementia.

WHAT HAPPENS AFTER THE MEDICAL ASSESSMENT

In most states, this is the sequence of events if the physicians find that any of the above criteria apply to the patient's situation:

- They issue a "2PC," a two-physician certificate.
- The certificate is taken immediately to a judge (these judges are on call twenty-four hours a day) while the patient is still in the emergency room.
- In general, the judges concur with the physician's assessment. The patient will be sent to a psychiatric hospital. A follow-up medical assessement, and a second review by a judge, must take place seventy-two hours after the initial examination.

A Tough Decision Made Out of Concern

There is no way around the fact that the decision to call the rescue squad or the police is a difficult one, fraught with high emotion. You know, however, that if you've reached the point where this is the decision you must make, it's in your loved one's very best interest to act. Their very safety depends on it. It's better for you to do this, and to be there with the patient, than to have it done by a stranger who finds your loved one wandering along a highway in his pajamas at six a.m. in twenty-degree weather, or in some other such situation.

Concern, care, love—these are the factors behind commitment.

SIX

THE DIAGNOSTIC PROCESS

Differential diagnosis is the term doctors use to describe the diseases a person may have as exactly as possible. The plural word "diseases" is important since someone's dementia may have more than one cause.

In reading Chapter Three, you've seen that dementia can have a wide variety of causes. Further, as you've seen in several anecdotes, the patient history gives invaluable information to an experienced doctor diagnosing a patient with the symptoms of dementia.

As you can well understand, the compiling of the patient history is somewhat out of the ordinary when the person to be diagnosed has a memory disorder. Your father may not now remember having told you years earlier that his grandmother, who lived with his family, was "senile" in her later years—but you and your siblings do. Your parents still have the clippings about your uncle's glorious career as a Golden Gloves boxer—in the 1940s!—though he wouldn't know to mention that to a doctor looking into his Alzheimer's-like symptoms.

In short, the patient history, so vital to diagnosis, is

going to depend on your getting together with other family members—siblings, cousins, aunts, and uncles—to put together the information that will so help the doctor in the diagnostic process.

WHAT KIND OF INFORMATION IS INCLUDED IN THE PATIENT HISTORY?

The patient history includes the whole range of information relevant to diagnosing someone with dementia. These are the kinds of questions that would be asked:

- How did the condition manifest?
- Is there a history of what used to be called senility in the family?
- What other conditions run in the family?
- What medications, both prescription and over-the-counter, is the patient taking?
- Did the patient chronically abuse alcohol (even if such abuse took place years ago)?
- What medical conditions does the patient have (e.g., diabetes, high blood pressure)?
- Is there Lyme disease where the patient lives (or where the patient has traveled)?

PREPARING A PATIENT HISTORY AT HOME BEFORE YOUR FIRST DOCTOR'S APPOINTMENT

These in-depth questions will help you put together an informative patient history before your first appointment:

1. How did you (and possibly the patient) come to realize that something was wrong? Looking back, do
   you see that the memory problem came on slowly
   over a period of years (a process referred to as "in-
   sidious" by doctors) or more quickly than that?

   Have physical problems developed as well? For
   instance, is the patient's speech slurred at times, or
   does he or she have trouble pronouncing words that
   formerly posed no problem? Are there difficulties in
   walking (what doctors would call gait disturbances)
   or standing (a station disturbance)?

2. Is there a history of "senility" on the patient's side
   of the family? Or is there perhaps a history of heart
   disease and/or stroke? Or of Parkinson's or Huntington's?

3. What about the patient's individual medical history?
   You'll recall from two cases presented in Chapter
   Three that aspects of the patients' medical history
   were vital clues to their doctors' arriving at the correct diagnosis. The retired engineer who turned out
   to have medication-induced dementia had been taking Valium, along with other medications, for twenty
   years, ever since he'd had a heart attack in his early
   fifties. The retired teacher had a mixed dementia
   (vascular dementia combined with a reversible condition, the pseudodementia caused by depression).
   The medical history revealed that she had experienced three prior depressions in her life.

   Did the patient chronically abuse alcohol, even in
   the past?

   Does he or she have high blood pressure, or high
   cholesterol or triglyceride levels?

   Has the patient ever had a blood transfusion?

   Does the patient have diabetes?

What medications is the patient taking, prescription and over-the-counter?

What about the patient's nutrition?

- Is he or she eating balanced meals?
- Have any cravings, such as for sweets, developed?
- Have there been any other changes in his or her normal patterns of eating (eating much more frequently, for example)?

Any changes in sleep patterns? If so, what are they (falling asleep much earlier or later, awakening much earlier or oversleeping)?

4. What about past activities and/or places visited?

- Could the patient have been exposed to industrial toxins in the workplace?
- Was the patient involved in sports or activities that may have involved head trauma?
- Did he or she at any time suffer a severe blow to the head, perhaps in an accident or in falling from a height?
- Is there Lyme disease in the patient's neighborhood, or did the patient go to such an area in recent years?

5. Are there problems doing what he or she could do before (functional difficulties)? Has interest in previously enjoyed activities fallen off? Think about these areas:

- Paying bills/balancing a checkbook.
- Recalling *recent* events.

- Learning new things, such as how to work recently bought appliances or fresh information pertaining to a job or other activity.
- Recalling people once well known to the patient.
- Getting lost coming home, or in another familiar place.
- Games/activities of skill—chess, crossword puzzles, musical instruments, and the like.
- Other hobbies, such as gardening or collecting.

6. Differences in behavior and personality. Think about these areas:

- Level of hostility or apathy—has it increased?
- Is there evidence of a depressed or hostile mood?
- Does the person exhibit signs of paranoia—claiming, for instance, that his grown children are trying to steal his money?
- Has a social person become more withdrawn lately?
- Has an already pleasant person become exceptionally nice and accommodating?
- Other changes from the person's norm, such as someone who always wore expensive clothing wearing much lower quality items that he or she wouldn't have before; other changes in taste or grooming.

A FINAL CHECK BEFORE YOU LEAVE FOR THAT FIRST APPOINTMENT

Make sure you have the following:

1. The patient history you and other family members, along with the patient, have prepared.
2. A list of all the drugs, both prescription and over-the-counter, that the patient is taking. Bring all prescription bottles with you. To keep them all in one place, you might want to put them in the type of plastic bag you get at a store to carry purchases.
3. The patient's recent previous medical records. For instance, if a chest X ray has been taken within the past few years, call the doctor who ordered it and bring a copy to your first appointment; do the same for other records, such as the result of blood tests or other tests taken in the past few years. If you're having trouble getting all those records, however, don't let that delay your dealing with the memory disorder. This is an important, current issue, and it has to be addressed—the sooner it is, the sooner you and your family can take further action to help your loved one.

IN THE DOCTOR'S OFFICE: TWO ALL-IMPORTANT MEDICAL TESTS TO START THE DIAGNOSTIC PROCESS

Sometimes we can overlook the simple and obvious as we struggle to deal with the complexity of memory disorders. Our situation can be similar to those times when an appliance wasn't working, and we tried all sorts of complicated ways to fix it, only to realize it wasn't plugged in. That's the kind of experience two vital medical tests can address.

What are they? Tests of vision and hearing.

For a variety of reasons, older people experiencing a

decline in these two senses won't—or can't—take care of the problem. Sometimes they don't take action because the decline, while steady, is slow and unnoticeable on a daily, weekly, or even monthly basis. Or those who are, indeed, in the earlier stages of a memory disorder are often no longer able to cope with this level of personal caretaking.

HOW VISION AND HEARING PROBLEMS CAN AFFECT PEOPLE

Problems in these two areas can make a memory disorder seem worse, and they greatly add to the sufferer's isolation and discomfort—and increase frustration for caregivers. It is common for many of those who are losing their hearing to refuse to acknowlege the fact, and adapt strategies to conceal their loss from others. For instance, in order not to have to respond to words they are likely not to understand, some people cope with hearing loss by dominating conversations, giving no one else a chance to speak. Or their misunderstanding questions or the general line of a conversation will make them respond inappropriately, and they can seem more confused than they actually are.

A thorough medical exam will include a basic assessment of hearing and vision. And while it's easy to start using new glasses (all you have to do now is keep track of them!), it can be more frustrating but ultimately very rewarding to cope with hearing loss. Keep at it until you find the hearing aid that works best for the person. Use other strategies such as speaking more slowly and distinctly, and let the person see your face when you speak—it's much easier to interpret the words that way. If necessary, communicate in writing, especially when you wish to convey important information clearly.

ON TO THE REST OF THE DIAGNOSIS

Earlier in this chapter, you read about a full range of areas to consider before the first visit to the doctor. Remember, in assessing someone showing the symptoms of dementia, doctors have to rely on other family members more than they do when examining those not suffering memory impairment.

In taking the patient history, doctors will first ask what has brought you to the office to begin with; that is, what symptoms is the person showing? In the cause of dementia, these include memory problems first and foremost, but possibly also problems with speech, changes in walking or standing (gait and station disturbances), noticeable changes in sleep or eating patterns, possibly hallucinations and/or noticeable changes in personality.

The physician will then ask about the onset of the reported symptoms. Was there a gradual deterioration of the patient's ability to remember, to think clearly and logically, to handle the functions of everyday life? And if so, how gradual? Did it take years for others to notice the problems that have brought you to the doctor's office, or was the decline faster and therefore more readily noticeable, taking place over months rather than years, and perhaps following the steplike decrease in ability that often signals vascular dementia?

Other questions physicians will ask in taking the patient history include:

- What medical conditions does the patient currently have, and what medications, both prescription and over-the-counter, is the patient taking?
- What about the patient's earlier medical history? Is there, for example, a history of high blood pressure, heart disease, depression, or alcohol abuse? Has the patient ever had blood transfusions? Or head injuries? And, since the advent of the woman boxer is only just upon us, did *he* box as a young man?
- Family medical history—did any relatives have what used to be called senility? Or heart disease or strokes, or perhaps Parkinson's or Huntington's disease? Have any of the patient's siblings been diagnosed with these conditions?
- Any changes in what physicians refer to as "appetitive functions," sleep, eating, and sexual interest and performance?
- What about changes in executive function, the ability to plan and carry out activities that once gave the patient no trouble? What about skills the patient could once perform and now can no longer, from balancing a checkbook to playing chess to figuring out answers on "Wheel of Fortune"?
- Any changes in sociability or personality?
- What about the possibility of Lyme disease? Does the patient live in one of the many areas in the country where the disease exists, or did she or he travel to such an area before the onset of symptoms?

A MENTAL STATUS EXAM

This is also called a *psychiatric exam*, and is performed by a physician who is experienced in the diagnosis of memory disorders, usually a neurologist, a psychiatrist, or a geriatrician (a physician who specializes in the care of older people). It is an assessment of general appearance and behavior, including a series of questions that reveal the patient's orientation to time, place, and other people (e.g., does he know where he is right now, what day and year it is, and his relation to the people who have accompanied him to the appointment?); the patient's mood; how the patient thinks and speaks; and the patient's cognitive functioning—memory and the capacity for abstract thought, insight, and judgment. The patient is asked, for instance, how he or she would handle certain situations, such as finding a wallet in the street. The patient is also asked to perform such tasks as spelling words backwards, and counting backwards from a certain number.

There are two standardized exams of mental status, both marked on a numbered scale. They are usually administered by the physician in the office, and are:

1. *The Mental Status Questionnaire (MSQ)*—The MSQ is comprised of ten questions pertaining to the patient's date of birth, the current date and day, where he or she currently is, and questions about the current president and past presidents.
2. *The Mini-Mental State Examination (MMSE)*—The MMSE contains the same type of questions pertaining to dates and locations as does the MSQ, but also tests more complex functions such as arithmetic skills, ability to visualize and draw a design, and tests of both long- and short-term memory. Being more in-depth, it gives a more complete indication of the patient's state than the MSQ.

THE PHYSICAL EXAM

This is the part of the exam with which we're all familiar, those assessments that are part of any physical, such as height, weight, and blood pressure. Other aspects include evaluation of the body's systems, such as cardiovascular, gastrointestinal, and pulmonary. As noted earlier in this chapter, a good physical will ideally include basic tests of vision and hearing.

A THOROUGH NEUROLOGIC EXAM

This involves observation as well as the laying on of hands by the physician. It is an evaluation of the peripheral and the central nervous systems (the brain and the spinal cord), and includes several assessments, such as testing of motor function (for example, how well does the person walk?), sensory perception, reflexes, and involuntary movement such as tremors. The exam combines trained observation with clinical skills on the part of the physician.

BLOOD WORK

The following blood tests may be given:

CBC (complete blood count)—to look for anemia and infections
sedimentation rate—to look for inflammation and infections
electrolytes—to check for salts, such as sodium and potassium

BUN/creatinine—to check kidney function
liver function tests
calcium
thyroid function tests ·
serum B_{12} level
syphilis serology
HIV testing
testing for Lyme disease

EKG

The electrocardiogram (ECG, EKG) tests for abnormalities of the heart.

URINALYSIS

A physical, microscopic, or chemical examination of urine. It may reveal such signs of illness as pus or bacteria, and/or quantify the presence of such substances as sugar, protein, ketones, or blood in the urine.

NEUROIMAGING STUDIES

The advent of the CT and MRI scans of the head revolutionized diagnosis of dementia, since they reveal many potentially treatable conditions that would otherwise be missed: tumors, subdural hematomas, hydrocephalus, and strokes.

The *CT scan—computerized tomography* (originally known as the CAT scan, for computerized axial tomography). It reveals gross structural changes to the brain through greater sensitivity to brain tissue density than the standard X ray. It will show most brain tumors, and is especially good at revealing the series of small strokes known as multi-infarct dementia (one of the vascular dementias). In fact, it is much more useful in the diagnosis of these strokes than it is in the diagnosis of Alzheimer's.

The *MRI—magnetic resonance imaging.* The MRI reveals cerebral infarcts, tumors, hemorrhages, and vascular abnormalities, as well as any possible atrophy (shrinking) of the brain.

Two newer brain scans may also be used in diagnosis. They are the *PET scan* (for *positron-emission tomography*) and the *SPECT scan* (for *single-photon-emission computed tomography*). Whereas the CT and MRI scans show *structure* of the brain, PET and SPECT scans provide information about cerebral *function,* about the metabolism of the brain. They show where function in the brain appears to be altered in ways now associated with Alzheimer's. While the PET scan has more resolution and sensitivity than the SPECT scan, the SPECT scan is less expensive and more readily available.

FORMAL NEUROPSYCHOLOGICAL TESTING

These are standardized, specific formats and tests usually administered by a psychologist. Although not a requirement, they are often a useful adjunct in the diagnostic process. They are:

To estimate pre-illness verbal abilities:

The New Adult Reading Test

To test attention and executive function:

The Wechsler Adult Intelligence Scale—Revised
   trail making

To test motor ability:

grooved peg-Board
finger tapping

To test language:

The Boston Naming Test
The verbal fluency test

To test visuospatial/constructional abilities:

WAIS-R Block Design
The Hooper Visual Organization Test

To test memory:

The Wechsler Memory Scale—Revised
The California Verbal Learning Test
The Blessed Information-Memory-Concentration
   Test
The Blessed Dementia Scale

To test personality and emotional functioning:

The MMPI-2 (the Minnesota Multi-phasic
   Inventory-2)

To assess activities of daily living:

The Outpatient Disability Scale of Pfeffer et al.

To differentiate between primary degenerative dementia and vascular dementia:

The Hachinski Ischemic Scale (especially as modified by Rosen et al.)

To diagnose depression and determine its severity:

The Beck Scale
The Hamilton Scale

There are two caveats to mention when discussing these tests. First, age, education, ethnic background, and language of the person being tested have all been shown to influence his or her responses; the doctor must make allowances for these factors in administering these tests. Also, a person who is very high functioning but who has noticed a decline in memory and other intellectual functions may indeed still score high enough on many of these tests not to show impairment. Such an individual should be tested again in about six months, so the doctor can assess whether a decline has taken place between test periods.

BEHAVIORAL TESTS

Part of the diagnostic process is determining just how much the dementia has impeded the patient's ability to function in daily life. The test given to show this is called *activities of daily living (ADL)*. The ADL assesses competence in a variety of areas. The first three pertain to daily activities, the last three to more complex behaviors linked to daily life:

1. Hygiene: Is the patient still able to groom himself, brush his teeth, bathe, change clothes?
2. Household tasks: Does he or she still do what was done in the past—set the table, fill the dishwasher, vacuum, dust, do the laundry?
3. Problem solving: Can he make up a shopping list? Does she note household repairs to be done, then fix them or arrange for them to be fixed?
4. Financial: Can he or she still handle money accurately? If the patient handled family finances in the past—paid bills, kept the household checkbook—can he or she still do this?
5. Social: Can the patient still participate socially at his or her earlier level? How is one-on-one interaction, small-group interaction, large-group interaction? Can he or she still perform earlier, skilled social activities such as card games, chess, Scrabble?
6. Personal: Is the person still concerned about others, still showing previous levels of respect toward others? Can he or she control emotions appropriately?

The ADL enables the family to assess the sorts of changes that have taken place in the patient, and to better understand future changes as they occur.

SOME OPTIONAL TESTS

Lumbar puncture (spinal tap)—tests the fluids that bathe the brain; generally not useful in diagnosing dementia in elderly patients. This test is recommended under certain conditions, including when the person with dementia is under fifty-five, or when there has been a rapidly progressive or unusual dementia.

EEG (electroencephalogram)—a noninvasive measure of the brain's electrical activity. This test is not recommended as a routine study, but may be useful in distinguishing dementia from depression or delirium, in revealing seizures as a cause of memory loss, or in evaluating for suspected encephalitis, Creutzfeldt-Jakob disease, or metabolic encephalopathy.

DIAGNOSIS ITSELF: WHAT IT SHOULD MEAN

At last! The entire diagnostic process has been completed, and you are now to be told the patient's diagnosis.

It's important to keep in mind that a diagnosis is not merely a label. It should:

- Give you information about the underlying cause (or causes) of symptoms.
- Indicate what should be done to alleviate those symptoms.
- Provide you with information about how to proceed, both in terms of medical treatments (discussed in the next chapter) *and* other implications of the particular diagnosis—referrals to such appropriate sources as support organizations and those county and state offices that provide information about social services (discussed in Chapter Eight).

An example of an ideal diagnosis is the one a family received at a suburban hospital-affiliated memory disorder center in a county neighboring theirs. The physician who directed the center presented the diagnosis, discussed its implications, and referred the family to a protocol being led by a nearby physician. This was before any Alzheimer's-specific drugs had been approved by the FDA, and the particular protocol was for tacrine, which eventually was marketed as Cognex, the first FDA-approved drug developed to treat Alzheimer's. The director of the center then turned the meeting over to a geriatric nurse and a social worker, who had been present from the start. They gave the family further information, including resources in their county, even though the center was in another county. Of course, the family was to phone any of the three if more questions arose later.

You can readily see the value of such a thorough approach to diagnosis. Do not stop with diagnoses that do not provide the preceding information. Considering what is now known about memory disorders, particularly the growth of knowledge about Alzheimer's alone in the past few years, a diagnosis that simply names the disease is not enough.

If your doctor cannot speak with you about the cause and probable progression of the disease, as well as about treatments and other services, you need to find a doctor who can. See Chapter Four for information.

SO NOW YOU HAVE A DIAGNOSIS: THE NEXT STAGE OF LIFE BEGINS

In the remaining chapters of this book, you'll be reading about such topics as coping with everyday living with an Alzheimer's patient, finding an adult day center, and learning what the future in general holds.

First, however, you'll be reading about the next thing you should be attending to—the medical treatment of your loved one.

SEVEN

TREATMENT OPTIONS

One of the best aspects of the fight against Alzheimer's is the progress made in recent years in treating patients. One of the saddest is that most people, among them many doctors, are not aware of the range of treatments, or even that Alzheimer's can be treated at all.

This lack of awareness means that you may well have to be the driving force behind getting treatment for the patient. Similar to getting a diagnosis, this may be difficult and frustrating at times. But when you've succeeded, it can be very rewarding.

Knowing a loved one's well-being was at stake kept you going during trying times in seeking a diagnosis. Now keep in mind that everyone with Alzheimer's can benefit from treatment, with, at the least, the patient being made more comfortable. At best, they can work very well, giving your family more, and more enjoyable, time with your loved one.

Seeking Treatment Can be Like Seeking a Diagnosis . . .

In the quest for a diagnosis, you had to be resourceful and persistant. You also had to be informed, about symptoms, networking, diagnosis, getting people to cooperate. Now you're on another quest, to get the best possible treatment.

. . . Information Motivates Action

Again, you'll have to be resourceful and persistant. And you'll have to be informed, about treatments now available, about how they work, about drug protocols. Chapter Two presented the changes in the brain caused by the disease. Now you'll see how current treatments affect those changes. Understanding the way they work will help in the potentially frustrating task ahead; it can strengthen your resolve to find the best ones for the patient and help you get family members to cooperate.

THE CURRENT STATE OF TREATING ALZHEIMER'S

Since the disease is now better understood, treatments are better and patients are much more fortunate than those of even the recent past. Treatments fall into five categories:

1. Drugs developed specifically to treat aspects of the disease process; there are two such drugs.
2. Drugs developed to treat other conditions that affect the actual disease process and may benefit some pa-

tients; there are almost twenty such drugs.
3. Drugs that treat behavorial symptoms; there are over fifty such drugs.
4. Drugs not yet approved for any use by the FDA currently being studied in protocols to determine if they're safe and effective in treating Alzheimer's.
5. Food supplements, herbs, and vitamins.

Later in this chapter you'll find more information and lists of these treatments.

THE WAY DRUGS ARE CLASSIFED

Drugs are broken into three classifications:

1. **FDA approved**. These may be labeled, promoted, and advertised by the manufacturer only for those uses for which their safety and effectiveness have been established in double-blind, placebo-controlled studies. Only after extensive testing will the FDA consider approving drugs.
2. **Off label**. Using an FDA-approved drug for a purpose other than the one (or ones) for which it's been approved is an off-label use. For instance, though the approved use of the nicotine patch is to help people quit smoking, when doctors noticed that it seemed to help some patients with Alzheimer's, they used it to treat the disease. A study published in Fall 1996 showed why it may help—nicotine seems to prevent the formation of plaques in the brain. If protocols establish this as safe and effective, it would likely become an FDA-approved use.
   While the off-label use of drugs by physicians is

perfectly legal, some doctors do not like to do it.
You and the patient's doctor may find this to be a
point of contention; this kind of conflict is discussed
in Chapter Four.

3. **Experimental drugs**. These have not yet been approved by the FDA for any use though they are being tested in protocols. Some doctors actively
encourage patients to participate in protocols, which
can be appealing in a disease like Alzheimer's, since
the FDA has approval only two drugs specifically
for it and since the protocol pays all expense related
to participating. However, considering the range of
current treatments and the frequent restrictions on
participants' use of other drugs and large doses of
vitamins, a protocol is not always the best option.
Following is information that can help you decide.

DRUG PROTOCOLS—WHAT THEY ARE

The studies undertaken to determine if a drug is safe
and effective are called protocols. A double-blind,
placebo-controlled protocol, the most common, is the
gold standard of experiments, the most rigorous and
useful.

''Placebo-controlled'' means that some participants
are in the *control group*; they do not take the actual
drug, but instead receive a placebo, a harmless substi-
tute pill. The control group helps show the drug's effect
on those actually taking it, since some of them experience the *placebo effect* of the drug, the often beneficial
but usually temporary effect produced psychologically
in some taking the placebo. To be seen as effective, the
drug being studied must reveal a significantly better re-

sult than the placebo. Rigorous statistical measurements ensure a valid, reliable difference.

"Double blind" means that neither the doctors conducting the study nor the participants know who is getting the drug, who the placebo. This method reduces any psychological effect that a doctor's or patient's expectations may have on the patient.

Weighing The Risks and Benefits of Protocols

Further—and this is a vital point—to show that any effects of the studied drug are caused solely by it, in *the vast majority of protocols, participants may not take other drugs their doctors might normally prescribe, or large doses of vitamins.* These restrictions last the duration of the protocol, probably about six months. As in all treatment situations, you must weigh risks versus benefits, here potential benefits against recognized ones.

The nature of the studied drug would help in your decision. For instance, Cognex and Aricept work by inhibiting the breakdown of acetylcholine. Entering a protocol for another drug that does the same thing may promise little gain, unless you've already seen that the patient does not respond to the two approved drugs (those who do not respond to one drug in a specific class and mechanism of action may respond to another one; for example, while the antidepressants Prozac and Paxil both inhibit the re-uptake of the neurotransmitter serotonin, some respond to one and not the other).

Since the earlier that certain treatments are prescribed the better their effect, time is also an important consideration. As it's recognized that treatments like Cognex, Aricept, nicotine, and vitamin E may slow the progression of the disease, do you want to risk that benefit to be in a protocol?

Discuss these important medical considerations with an experienced doctor. You and other family members should make the decision that makes you feel most comfortable.

How to Find Out About Drug Protocols

The Alzheimer's Association provides drug fact sheets on all nationwide protocols currently open (still taking participants). To get them phone 1-800-272-3900. Local chapters have information on regional protocols. Another way to find out about these is to get association drug sheets on nationwide protocols and check the ''Where will the studies take place?'' section. Call nearby centers listed to learn about other protocols being conducted there.

REVIEWING THE BASICS:
THE WAY ALZHEIMER'S AFFECTS
THE BRAIN

Seeing how treatments act on the effects of Alzheimer's can help you persevere in seeking them. Discussed in depth in Chapter Two, the major changes of Alzheimer's on the brain are:

1. A decreased level of acetylcholine.
2. The formation of plaques and tangles.
3. Damage to and the death of neurons, notably the cholinergic neurons vital to producing acetylcholine.
4. Problems in the process called glucose metabolism.

5. Damage to the mitochondria, vital to energy production.

Alzheimer's affects the brain in other ways that respond to treatment, notably decreasing levels of other neurotransmitters, including serotonin, norepinephrine, and dopamine (treatable by antidepressants). Free radicals (treated by antioxidants) also can damage neurons, as can inflammation (anti-inflammtory drugs may be of benefit).

TREATMENTS FOR ALZHEIMER'S

An important caveat regarding the use of all treatments. Many of the following drugs are available only by prescription, so their use is supervised by a qualified physician. Yet several drugs and all of the food supplements and vitamins are available without a prescription. These are potent substances on their own, and they may interact in unpredictable—and dangerous—ways. Use the following treatments *only* under the supervision of an experienced physician.

Drugs approved specifically for treating Alzheimer's

Generic	Trade	Comments
donepezil	Aricept	no liver toxicity to date; once a day dosing
tacrine	Cognex	first approved; liver toxicity (in some cases); several times a day dosing

Cognex, approved in 1993, and Aricept, approved in 1997, work in the same way and address the decrease in acetylcholine by inhibiting acetylcholinesterase (also known simply as cholinesterase), the enzyme that breaks down acetylcholine.

The next generation of Cognex, Aricept requires fewer doses and does not have the potential to inflame the liver, as Cognex may. Both have similar side effects, which include diarrhea, nausea, and vomiting. If these side effects appear, they often abate or lessen in a few weeks. The effect of these drugs can be so beneficial that doctors may treat these side effects, if they occur, rather than stop the drug.

If prescribed early enough and in a high enough dosage, both may show an unexpected, beneficial secondary effect, one that addresses plaque formation in the brain. In an interview in the October 1997 *Psychiatric Times*, leading researcher Ken Davis, M.D., notes that, by stimulating the cholinergic system, they in some way decrease the production of harmful a-beta (a component of plaques). He says that by doing so these drugs, "may actually alter the course of the disease, in addition to simply improving symptoms." A beneficial effect indeed, and one that may lead to further treatments.

SOME OFF-LABEL DRUGS THAT MAY BENEFIT ALZHEIMER'S PATIENTS

Generic	Trade	Comment
aspirin		anti-inflammatory

bromocriptine	Parlodel	antiparkinson agent
buproprion	Wellbutrin	antidepressant
dehydroepiandrosterone (DHEA)		steroid hormone
estrogen		female hormone
fluoxetine	Prozac	antidepressant
hydergine		general cognitive enhancer (used in high doses in Europe)
ibuprofen	Motrin, etc.	anti-inflammatory (other anti-inflammatories may be helpful, e.g., aspirin)
nicotine patch	Nicoderm, etc.	smoking cessation
nimodipine	Nimotop	calcium channel blocker used for hypertension
paroxetine	Paxil	antidepressant
pergolide	Permax	antiparkinson
physostigmine	Antilirium	increases acetylcholine (used to treat certain acute confusional states induced by other drugs)

Generic	Trade	Comment
prednisone		anti-inflammatory hormone
selegiline	Eldepryl	antiparkinson
sertraline	Zoloft	antidepressant
venlafaxine	Effexor	antidepressant
yohimbine	Yocon	sexual stimulant

Eighteen distinct drugs are listed above; most can be grouped into the following types: hormones (dehydroepiandrostefone and estrogen), antiparkinson drugs (Eldepryl, Parlodel, and Permax), antidepressant drugs (Paxil, Prozac, Wellbutrin, and Zoloft), and anti-inflammatory drugs (aspirin, ibuprofen, and prednisone). Of the remaining five, Antilirium blocks anticholinergic medications taken in purposeful or inadvertant overdose, Hydergine is a cognitive enhancer, the nicotine patch is a drug developed to aid in smoking cessation, Nimotop is an antihypertensive, and Yocon is a sexual stimulant.

All of these drugs are FDA-approved, though the treatment of Alzheimer's is currently an off-label use of all of them. Several of the drugs are being studied now specifically for their safety and efficacy in treating Alzheimer's, which may become an additional FDA-approved use of some of them.

HOW DRUGS DEVELOPED TO TREAT OTHER DISEASES HELP SOME ALZHEIMER'S PATIENTS

Why have these drugs shown to be useful in treating some people with Alzheimer's? Some of the reasons for their usefulness are not entirely understood; as noted in the previous section, Cognex and Aricept did what they were designed to do, which was inhibit the breakdown of acetylcholine, and also had the unexpected secondary good effect of decreasing the production of a-beta and therefore of amyloid plaques. And you will recall reading that several physicians had noticed that the nicotine patch helped some Alzheimer's patients, so they started to use it to treat the disease. Only in autumn 1996 did they learn why this beneficial effect might exist, when a study reporting that nicotine seems to stop the formation of amyloid plaques was published.

It is known why most of these drugs help treat Alzheimer's, or at least one or some of the reasons are known; research may reveal secondary good effects of any or all of them. As noted previously, your understanding why they work will underscore their value to you and help you persevere in seeking the right treatments for your loved one with Alzheimer's. In the following information, reference will be made to the numbered list of effects of Alzheimer's on the brain which appears earlier in this chapter.

Hormones (dehydroepiandrosterone and estrogen)

Dehydroepiandrosterone is the most abundant steroid hormone in the bloodstream, and brain tissue contains over six times the amount found in the bloodstream; it is believed that such high levels of DHEA protect the brain from the damage of aging. While everyone's level of DHEA decreases with age, the decrease is especially severe in Alzheimer's patients; they have only half of the amount in non-Alzheimer's patients of the same age. DHEA probably affects the brain in a similar way to estrogen, protecting cholinergic neurons and therefore dealing with points one and three of the listed effects of Alzheimer's on the brain, decreased levels of acetylcholine and damage to cholinergic neurons.

n   To repeat an important caveat—classified as a food supplement rather than as a drug in the United States, DHEA has not had to meet FDA standards for safety and efficacy. Obviously, however, it is quite a potent drug; further, it is a hormone and its long-term side effects are not known. **Use DHEA and other over-the-counter substances** *only* **under the supervision of a doctor**.

Estrogen is known to nourish cholinergic neurons; it thereby addresses point three, damage to and the death of cholinergic neurons. Since these neurons produce acetylcholine, necessary to the production of acetylcholine, increasing their health also addresses point one, decreased levels of this vital neurostransmitter. Though not in common practice, some doctors use the estrogen patch to treat both men and women with Alzheimer's. The relationship between hormone replacement therapy (HRT) in women and Alzheimer's is currently being studied in a nationwide protocol, the Women's Health Initiative Memory Study (WHI-MS) of Estrogen and Alzheimer's Disease, an ancillary study of the fifteen-year Women's Health Initiative. All participants entering this protocol are between the ages of sixty-five and seventy-nine; the study is currently scheduled to conclude in 2002, but may be extended until 2005. Data from all studies comprising the Women's Health Initiative are to be published in 2007.

Estrogen and Alzheimer's:
An Additional Consideration for Women Thinking
About Hormone Replacement Therapy

Considerable excitement has been generated however, concerning the potential of HRT to prevent or significantly slow the onset of Alzheimer's in women. Researchers including Anna Paginni-Hill, Ph.D., of UCLA and Claudia Kawas, M.D., of Johns Hopkins have reported promising information about HRT as an Alzheimer's preventitive to some women shown in retrospective studies. (By the way, in the early days of hormone replacement in menopausal women, the mid-1960s, estrogen alone was used, and the therapy was called estrogen replacement therapy, or ERT. Estrogen alone caused too great a risk of endometrial cancer (cancer of the endometrium, the lining of the uterus); precribing progesterone along with estrogen significantly reduced this risk, and the term hormone replacement therapy, or HRT, was born.)

This information about estrogen and Alzheimer's adds another element to the discussion of her family medical history any woman considering hormone replacement therapy would have with her doctor. While hormone replacement therapy has been shown to reduce symptoms of menopause such as hot flashes, and to prevent heart disease and osteoporosis in post-menopausal women, it increases the risk of breast cancer, and women using estrogen alone have an increased risk of endometrial cancer. (There is optimism that a "designer" estrogen called Evista (raloxifene), currently being studied and possibly available in the United States in the next few years, will not causes these risks.)

Factors to discuss with the doctor in addition to family medical history are a personal history of either breast or endometrial cancer, of undiagnosed abnormal vaginal bleeding or of liver dysfunction. Other factors which indicate that a woman may not be a good candidate for HRT are sickle cell disease, migraine headaches, uterine fibroids, gallbladder disease, and vascular disorders (blood vessel diseases such as hypertension).

Women with these factors in their personal medical history, as well as women who do not feel comfortable taking synthetic hormones for whatever reason, should discuss the use of *phytoestrogens*, or plant estrogens, with a qualified physician or dietician. Phytoestrogens seem to block the cancer-stimulating effect of estrogen, but whether they must be taken with a certain amount of fiber in the diet to have this effect has not yet been fully investigated. Phytoestrogens are also antioxidants. They can be found in the following foods:

   Soybeans and soy products (tofu, soy milk)
   Flax seeds, whole grains, sunflower seeds
   Apples, strawberries, grapes, pears, plums
   Cabbage, carrots, broccoli, tomatoes, garlic,
      squash

All types of estrogen are hormones; their use must be supervised by a qualified physician.

Antiparkinson Drugs (Parlodel, Permax, and Eldepryl)

Alzheimer's has shown some similarities to Parkinson's Disease, a significant one being damage to the mitochondria, point five. These antiParkinson drugs are antioxidants and address damage to the mitochondria. Eldepryl also inhibits the breakdown of dopamine.

In April of 1997 the *New England Journal of Medicine* reported a study of 10mg/day of selegiline (Eldepryl) and 2,000 international units (i.u.'s) of vitamin E, separately and combined, as treatments for Alzheimer's. Use of vitamin E alone showed the best results in delaying progress of the disease, followed closely by the use of selegiline alone. More information about vitamin E appears in the section in which food suppplements and vitamins are discussed.

Antidepressant Drugs (Paxil, Prozac, Wellbutrin, Zoloft, et al.)

As noted immediately following the list of five major effects of Alzheimer's on the brain, acetylcholine is not the only neurotransmitter that shows decreased levels in Alzheimer's. Levels of others such as serotonin, norepinephrine, and dopamine also decrease. Wellbutrin increases levels of norepinephrine and dopamine, Prozac, Paxil, and Zoloft increase levels of serotonin. Many other antidepressants act on these neurotransmitters.

Anti-inflammatory Drugs (aspirin, ibuprofen, and prednisone)

Also as noted immediately following the list of five major effects of Alzheimer's on the brain, inflammation is the cause of some of the damage to cells during the disease process. Currently being studied in low doses as an Alzheimer's treatment at Mount Sinai School of Medicine in New York, prednisone is a steroid hormone with powerful anti-inflammatory properties. It is a prescription drug which a number of physicians have found to be of benefit to some of their Alzheimer's patients. Aspirin and ibuprofen are non-steroidal anti-inflammatory drugs (NSAI's). Retrospective studies of arthritis patients who took significant amounts of aspirin and/or ibuprofen daily for years showed that fewer of these people developed Alzheimer's than did others of comparable age. These were tremendous amounts of ibuprofen and/or aspirin, however, taken daily to counter the effects of a debilitating disease; since these two drugs are such regular inhabitants of our home medicine cabinet it's easy to forget how potent they are, especially in high doses. They can cause bleeding in the stomach and kidney problems. **Do not start giving an Alzheimer's patient large amounts of ibuprofen or aspirin, or start taking large amounts yourself as a preventive measure; only a qualified physician can determine what drugs, in what quantities, are safest and most useful.**

Antilirium (physotigmine)

This drug blocks anticholinergic medications taken in purposeful or inadvertant overdose. Anticholinergic drugs include Cogentin (benztropine) used in Parkinson's and tricyclic antidepressants such as Tofranil (imipramine). By reversing anticholinergic effects, it increases cholinergic activity and levels of acetylcholine. Unfortunately, Antilirium can only be used intravenously and its effects on Alzheimer's disappear quickly. It is hoped that someday a long acting or oral preparation will be available.

Hydergine

In a study led by Branconnier and published in 1983, Hydergine was shown to be the first drug that could have beneficial effects on some Alzheimer's patients. These properties of the drug are believed to be among the reasons for this effect: in addition to lowering blood pressure and thereby improving the flow of blood to and within the brain, Hydergine has anti-oxidant properties, so it can affect damage to cholinergic neurons and to mitochondria. It also mimics in some way a substance called nerve growth factor (NGF), which affects the growth of dendrites, the part of neurons involved in receiving the signals carried by neurotransmitters. Hydergine is used in much higher doses in Europe than in the United States. It has met with mixed reviews in studies over the years.

The Nicotine Patch

As noted previously, some doctors noticed that the nicotine patch was of benefit to some Alzheimer's patients several years prior to the late 1996 publication of a study that showed that nicotine helped prevent the formation of amyloid plaques in the brain. It is not yet known how nicotine does this; perhaps, like Cognex and Aricept, by stimulating cholinergic activity it somehow affects the production of harmful a-beta, a necessary component of the plaques.

Nimotop (nimodipine)

Developed to treat high blood pressure, Nimotop improves the flow of blood to and within the brain. As a calcium channel blocker however, Nimotop probably also benefits some Alzheimer's patients by affecting the uncontrolled and potentially fatal flow of calcium into damaged neurons. It is interesting to note that Hydergine, described in the chart as a cognitive enhancer, was originally developed as an antihypertensive drug and was the first drug shown in a study to have some beneficial effects on Alzheimer's. It is discussed in more detail later in this section.

Yocon (yohimbine)

A sexual stimulant derived from the bark of the yohimbine tree, and used initially to treat male impotence, Yocon has been of benefit to some Alzheimer's patients. It increases levels of acetylcholine and norepiphrine.

SOME DRUGS USED FOR BEHAVIORAL SYMPTOMS OF ALZHEIMER'S DISEASE AND OTHER DEMENTIAS

Symptom	Chemical Name	Trade (Brand) Name
Anxiety	buspirone	Buspar
	clonazepam	Klonopin
	lorazepam	Ativan
	oxazepam	Serax
Insomnia	chlorpromazine	Thorazine
	clonazepam	Klonopin

estazolam	Prosom
lorazepam	Ativan
temazepam	Restoril
trazodone	Desyrel
thioridazine	Mellaril
zolpidem	Ambien

Depression

amphetamine	Dexedrine
buproprion	Wellbutrin
desipramine	Norpramin
doxepin	Sinequan
fluoxetine	Prozac
fluvoxamine	Luvox
methylphenidate	Ritalin
mirtazapine	Remeron
nefazadone	Serzone
nortriptyline	Pamelor
paroxetine	Paxil
sertraline	Zoloft
trazodone	Desyrel
trimipramine	Surmontil
venlafaxine	Effexor

Agitation

Major Tranquilizers:

chlorpromazine	Thorazine
haloperidol	Haldol
molindone	Moban
olanzepine	Zyprexa

Symptom	Chemical Name	Trade (Brand) Name
	risperidone	Risperdal
	thioridazine	Mellaril
	thiothixene	Navane
	Others:	
	buspirone	Buspar
	carbamazepine	Tegretol
	clonazepam	Klonopin
	lorazepam	Ativan
	lithium	Eskalith and others
	propranolol	Inderal
	divalproex	Depakote
Psychosis (Hallucinations/Delusions)		
	chlorpromazine	Thorazine
	haloperidol	Haldol
	molindone	Moban
	olanzepine	Zyprexa
	risperidone	Risperdal
	thioridazine	Mellaril
	Thiothixene	Navene

Other drugs discussed elsewhere in this chapter may have a beneficial effect on the behavioral symptoms of Alzheimer's, such as anxiety, insomnia, depression, agitiation, and psychosis (including hallucinations and delusions). Yet these symptoms are directly addressed and best managed by the drugs listed here, which have been approved by the FDA specifically to treat them.

The drugs used to treat psychiatric symptoms and disorders are called *psychotropics*. In patients with Alzheimer's and other dementias, psychotropics are complicated to use. First, symptoms must be accurately diagnosed in patients who often have difficulty communicating. In addition, since those with Alzheimer's have abnormalities in the functioning of the central nervous system, they are particularly sensitive to such drugs. Therefore psychotropics should be prescribed primarily by psychiatrists and at times by geriatricians or neurologists who have special expertise in using the drugs in Alzheimer's patients.

The use of these drugs is an extremely important aspect of treating Alzheimer's, since the vast majority of Alzheimer's patients will experience some of these symptoms during the course of the disease. Treating them appropriately is vital to seeing that the patient is made as comfortable as possible, and has a secondary effect; these treatable symptoms greatly affect not only the quality of life of the patient, but that of caregivers, and of the family as a whole. The relief provided enables them to cope better, and to better care for the patient.

SOME EXPERIMENTAL DRUGS BEING STUDIED FOR SAFETY AND EFFICACY IN TREATING ALZHEIMER'S

ampakine CX516 (Ampalex)
arecholine
ENA 713 (Exelon)
galanthamine

idebenone
metrifonate
milameline
nerve growth factor (NGF)
piracetam
propentofylline (HWA 285)

All of these experimental drugs are available only to those participating in protocols assessing their safety and efficacy. Protocols, the highly regulated studies in which the safety and efficacy of drugs is assessed, were discussed previously in this chapter; you will recall that all protocols have risks and benefits that must be discussed with the patient's doctor and carefully considered before the decision whether or not to participate is made. Contact the national Alzheimer's Association for information on nationwide protocols and the patient's local chapter to find out if any of the more limited protocols are being conducted nearby.

Following are brief descriptions of the experimental drugs listed in this category. You will note that several of them treat Alzheimer's in the same way that Cognex and Aricept do, by inhibiting the breakdown of acetylcholine. Keep in mind that people react differently to different drugs, and that one drug of this type may work very well in one person, and not in another; having several of them available increases treatment options for the Alzheimer's population as a whole.

Ampakine CX516 (Ampalex)

Newly developed compounds, ampakines are designed to enhance the functioning of AMPA-receptors.

These receptors respond to a neurotransmitter called glutamate and are believed to be vital to memory formation. Small studies have shown amapakine CX516 to enhance memory and learning in healthy adults; studies with Alzheimer's patients are just beginning.

Arecholine

Arecholine inhibits the breakdown of acetylcholine.

ENA 713 (Exelon)

ENA 713 inhibits the breakdown of acetylcholine and appears to be about to get FDA approval.

Galanthamine

Galanthamine inhibits the breakdown of acetylcholine.

Idebenone

Studies have already shown idebenone to improve memory, attention, and behavior in some Alzheimer's patients. It is believed to increase the brain's energy supply and increase the amount of nerve growth factor (NGF), which helps to protect against damage to neurons.

Metrifonate

Metrifonate inhibits the breakdown of acetylcholine.

Milameline

A drug that mimics the action of acetylcholine, milameline may effectively replace decreased amounts of this neurotransmitter in some Alzheimer's patients.

Nerve Growth Factor (NGF)

A protein found in the central nervous system that resembles insulin, nerve growth factor affects the growth and health of neurons.

Piracetam

Developed in Europe and used there to treat several conditions, piracetam is known as a cognitive enhancer; studies have shown it to enhance memory and learning in healthy people. One animal study has suggested that it may increase the number of cholinergic receptors in the brain, which may enable it to benefit some Alzheimer's patients.

Propentofylline (HWA 285)

Propentofylline seems to interrupt some of the factors that cause neurons to deteriorate and enhances cerebral blood flow and the metabolism of energy in the brain.

SOME FOOD SUPPLEMENTS, HERBS, AND VITAMINS THAT MAY BENEFIT SOME ALZHEIMER'S PATIENTS

acetyl-L-carnitine
choline
Co-enzyme Q-10
ginkgo biloba
lecithin
NADH
omega-3 fatty acids
Vitamin C
Vitamin E

No proof has yet been established regarding the usefulness of these food supplements and vitamins in treating some Alzheimer's patients, though some studies have shown promising results regarding the use of ginkgo biloba and vitamin E, which are still being studied, as are other substances in this category.

While all of these substances occur naturally and most are readily available in health food stores and some drug stores, it is vital to keep in mind that they work because they are powerful; further, they may interact with other substances being taken. Those using these substances should consult with a knowledgeable physician to ensure both safety and the best possible treatment.

A caveat regarding vitamin E and ginkgo: both may interfere with blood clotting and should be avoided or followed carefully by a physician in those taking an anticoagulant such as coumadin or in those with a history of hemophilia or other bleeding disorders. Those who take an aspirin a day as a heart attack preventitive generally do not have to be concerned with this precaution, though they should discuss the situation with their doctors.

A caveat regarding beta carotene: while most antioxidants have a beneficial effect, beta carotene should be avoided since current studies have reported contradictory information about its safety and effectiveness.

Following are brief descriptions of the substances listed in this category.

Acetyl-L-carnitine

A natural compound found in the body, acetyl-L-carnitine is involved in the normal functioning of mitochondria, which are damaged in Alzheimer's. Several studies in Italy have revealed some efficacy in slowing the progression of the disease. A current study is investigating whether acetyl-L-carnitine is more effective on those diagnosed with Alzheimer's between the ages of forty-five and sixty-five than on patients diagnosed after sixty-five.

Choline

The precusor of acetylcholine, choline improves memory by increasing the amount of this neurotransmitter.

Co-enzyme Q-10

This co-enzyme is vital to the mitochondria's production of energy. In addition to this role, co-enzyme Q-10 has anti-oxidant properties that protect neurons.

Ginkgo Biloba

Ginkgo biloba, an extract from the leaf of the ginkgo tree, has been used as a medicinal herb by the Chinese for thousands of years and has been widely prescribed in Europe in the past few decades to treat memory disorders. An anti-oxidant, ginkgo also reduces blood *viscosity*, or stickiness, thereby improving blood flow to and within the brain. Until recently, ginkgo had been shown to be effective in treating vascular dementia rather than Alzheimer's. However, a protocol reported in *The Journal of the American Medical Association (JAMA)* in October 1997 showed that a potent form of ginkgo could improve cognitive performance and social functioning in those with mild to moderate Alzheimer's. Participants took 40mg of the higher potency ginkgo three times a day. After six months, some participants demonstrated a modest benefit in cognitive performance and social functioning.

The high potency form of ginkgo tested in the study is EGb 761, the actual product name when gingko is prescribed in Germany. This same form of ginkgo is sold in the United States under the name GinkgolD by Nature's Way. Widely available in health food stores and other retail outlets, GinkgolD can also be ordered through the toll-free number of the parent company of Nature's Way, Murdock Madaus Schwabe, based in Springville, Utah. That number is 1-800-9-NATURE (1-800-962-8873).

Lecithin

A precursor to choline, lecithin is necessary in transforming fats in the body, and has as its active ingredient phosphatidyl choline, a form of choline which has some unique functions. As the source of material from which cell membranes are made it affects a number of neurochemical activities; it is also vital to the maintenance and repair of neurons, helps regulate cholesterol levels in the blood, and nourishes the sheaths of nerve fibers. Unfortunately, studies to date have not shown positive results in treating Alzheimer's; to achieve any kind of benefit, enormous quantities must be taken. Perhaps lecithin will become a better Alzheimer's treatment if a concentrated form is developed.

NADH

Similar to co-enzyme Q-10, NADH is a naturally occuring co-enzyme vital to the production of the neurotransmitter dopamine and to the energy producing process of the mitochondria. It has been shown to benefit some chronic fatigue syndrome patients in studies in Europe and its safety and efficacy in treating both chronic fatigue syndrome and Alzheimer's are currently being studied in protocols at Georgetown University Medical School.

Omega-3 fatty acids

An essential fatty acid found in such cold-water fish as salmon, mackerel, sardines, and herring, omega-3 fatty acids perform several vital functions in the body; a deficiency can cause damage to cells. Unfortunately, most Americans consume very low levels of omega-3 fatty acids. Adding cold-water fish to the diet and taking supplements can address this lack.

Vitamin C

An anti-oxidant, vitamin C protects against damage to cells by free radicals. It is a water-soluble vitamin, so any excess taken is excreted by the body. However, in very high doses it may have side effects and toxicity.

Vitamin E (alpha-tocopherol)

Vitamin E is a powerful anti-oxidant that has been shown to have a beneficial effect on some Alzheimer's patients. In April 1997 the *New England Journal of Medicine* reported a study of 10mg/day of selegiline (Eldepryl) and 2,000 international units (i.u.'s) of vitamin E, separately and combined, as treatments for Alzheimer's. Use of vitamin E alone showed the best results in delaying progress of the disease, followed closely by selegiline alone. A caution regarding vitamin E—it is a fat-soluble vitamin, so any excess taken will be retained by the body rather than excreted; further, as a fat-soluble vitamin, it must be taken with some fat in order to be absorbed. If taken with milk, a common option, the milk must be one percent fat or more; non-fat milk does not help in the absorbtion of vitamin E. The minimun daily is requirement is 400 i.u.'s; taking more should be discussed with your physician.

A Word About Prevention

Though the Alzheimer's disease process is not completely understood, it can certainly be treated in several ways. Proper, physician-supervised use of some of these treatments may also help slow the onset of Alzheimer's, important in a disease that appears late in life, or may even help prevent it.

As noted previously in this chapter in the discussion of estrogen, retrospective studies indicate that hormone replacement therapy may help slow the onset of Alzheimer's or possibly prevent it in women. And certainly a healthy diet including at minimum sufficient amounts of anti-oxidants, especially vitamin E and vitamin C, gingko biloba, fish that contain a lot of omega-3 fatty acids such as salmon and tuna, and other substances mentioned in the category of food supplements and vitamins could well have a beneficial preventive effect.

Further, cardiovascular fitness is extremely important to the health of the brain. Achieving it means reducing high blood pressure and having healthy levels of cholesterol and of triglycerides in the blood. Eating well figures strongly in this picture, as does physical exercise, a vital element in achieving and maintaining cardiovascular health.

Finally, exercising the brain itself may also prove beneficial. Try adding, subtracting, and multiplying using your brain rather than your calculator; keep phone numbers in your head rather than on speed dial (you will find this helpful if you find yourself at a pay phone without your address book); stretch your brain by doing crossword puzzles or other kinds of problems; think about doing some active writing rather than passive reading.

A final word about preventive strategies: similar to medications, effective as they may be for some people, not all work equally for everyone. Remember that Alzheimer's is a complicated disease process not fully understood. Also keep in mind that it's an illness, not a judgement. You may read that the better educated a person is, the less likely he or she is to develop Alzheimer's. While this may be true statistically, each individual is different. Alzheimer's patients include one of the first NASA rocket scientists as well as Sir Rudolph Bing, an internationally renowned wit who excelled in the demanding job of running New York's Metropolitan Opera. The fact that so many people develop Alzheimer's, and that the loss of each one affects the world in so many ways, only underlines the need to develop ever more effective treatments.

EIGHT

COPING WITH EVERYDAY LIFE:
STRATEGIES AND RESOURCES

Learning about the many medical treatments now available for Alzheimer's, which you did in Chapter Seven, is one of several immediate concerns when someone you know has been given a diagnosis of probable Alzheimer's. The others have to do with living with an Alzheimer's patient on a daily basis. You will be consulting more specialized sources for information about legal issues and finances, as that information varies from state to state and is subject to ever changing government regulations; in fact, advice in those areas should come from a qualified professional whom you have been referred to by others you trust. While you want to start investigating those issues as soon as possible, there are others that you must address right now. These all have to do with the physical and psychological safety of the Alzheimer's patient.

PATIENT SAFETY ISSUES—DRIVING, WANDERING, AND HOME SAFETY

Driving. We all know that a person whose dementia has progressed to a certain point is no longer capable of driving. Yet a recent study done in Scandinavia has shown that even those in the earlier stages of Alzheimer's are much more likely to have traffic accidents than they were before becoming ill. The issue of driving is, then, one to be addressed very soon after diagnosis, and it's an important one, involving not just the well-being of the patient, but of those on the road with him.

In most parts of our country, driving equals all things good—adulthood, independence, freedom. So caregivers must be aware of the importance of what the patient is being asked to give up, and consider a number of nonconfrontational techniques to prevent him or her from driving.

Many actions of those with Alzheimer's are triggered by direct stimulus, rather than by their planning in advance what they want to do, due to the deterioration of their executive, or planning, ability. So one tactic is not to park the family car (or cars) in its usual spot, where it can be readily seen from the house or yard. While parking the car around the corner can cause other family members some inconvenience, it can help you avoid many confrontations over this issue. In the same "out of sight, out of mind" vein, car keys should not be left out in open sight, since they inspire the desire to drive. Disabling the car, usually by removing spark plugs, is a technique that has worked for some. If the patient gets into the car and is not able to start it, the impulse to drive often falls away, with the patient not remembering where he intended to drive. Another technique, mentioned in the home safety guide we discuss in the "Home Safety" section in this chapter, is to ask the patient's doctor to write "Do Not Drive" on a prescription pad. This way, it's not just a family request that the patient not drive, but an official directive from the doctor.

Wandering. Wandering is a great danger to the safety of the patient, and is an equally great fear of the caregiver. We frequently hear about a demented person wandering away from a shopping trip, a local baseball game, or even from home itself at all hours of the day and night.

There are several systems for tracking wanderers. The most widely used, with twenty-eight thousand subscribers, is the Safe Return program of the Alzheimer's Association (1-800-272-3900). There is a $25 registration fee. Patients wear a bracelet or necklace featuring a toll-free number and their own Safe Return ID number. At the other end of the toll-free number is an operator who consults a computer database for the wanderer's identity.

Those registered in the Safe Return program also have identifying information about themselves entered into a national database; when someone is reported missing, information is then faxed about that person to area hospitals, shelters, and EMS services.

Starting in 1996, older people began to be registered on the Internet site Birthnet, originally designed for parents to register children in case they go missing. Adding adults to this service was the idea of nurse Marianne Dickerman Caldwell, who writes about her mother's wandering away from a softball game in the book *Gone Without a Trace* (available from Elder Books, whose books and other products are described in this chapter in "A Valuable Resource for Patient and Caregiver"). Law enforcement personnel, the media, and medical professionals can download identifying information about a wanderer.

Birthnet can be found on the Internet at http:// www.birthnet.com. There is no fee for a registry page. However, if you wish to feature a color photo of the loved one on the page, there is a fee of $12.95.

While several companies are investigating the feasibility of satellite tracking systems to locate wanderers, two firms in the United States offer transmitter tracking devices.

The receiving unit and search antenna of Care Track have been adopted by a number of law enforcement and rescue teams throughout the country. You can contact Care Track at 800-842-4537; renting their wrist transmitter and tracking device costs $35 a month, a fee reduced by $10 if you live near a police or rescue team using Care Track, as you then only have to rent the transmitter.

In addition to offering a wrist or ankle transmitter, which some Alzheimer's patients do not want to wear, Care Electronics of Colorado has a transmitter that can be embedded in a fanny pack, which is more acceptable to some patients. Instead of leasing its transmitter and tracking system, Care Electronics sells them for $775. The company can be reached at 303-444-2273.

Home Safety. Making the home safe for the Alzheimer's patient involves considering every room of the house. The very best source in this area is "Home Safety for the Alzheimer's Patient," a thirty-two-page brochure available in both English and Spanish from the Alzheimer's Disease Education and Referral Center

(ADEAR), for $2.50. You can send a check in that amount to:

The ADEAR Center
P.O. Box 8250
Silver Spring, MD 20907-8250
1-800-438-4380, 8:30 A.M. to 5:00 P.M. EST, Monday to Friday

ADULT DAY CENTERS

Whether the primary caregiver works outside the home or not, adult day services, also known as adult day care, can be a vital part of daily life for the Alzheimer's patient. Obviously, if you must be away from home during the day, you need to know that your loved one is safe and cared for, ideally having companionship and activities and getting both proper nutrition and medications on a timely basis. And if you stay at home during the day, having your loved one in a good day services program gives you some respite from the demands of caregiving. You'll also see that at the end of a day in such a setting, your loved one is usually more alert than on other days due to the stimulation received.

The growth in this area has been tremendous, as attested to by the increasing number of such centers listed in the various editions of The National Directory of Adult Day Care Centers, published by Health Resources Publishing. The first edition appeared in 1987 and listed 600 centers. That number had more than tripled by the time of the second edition in 1993, which listed almost 2,100 centers. The third edition, appearing in early 1998, features approximately 4,000 centers.

In addition to a center's name, address and phone number, an entry in the directory will list the name of the executive director, the date the program started, the type of ownership (corporate, partnership, private, etc.), whether the center is for profit or not, the type of model on which it's based, social (which cannot accommodate the medical needs of some attendees) or medical (with the staff to accommodate more medical needs than social centers can), services and activities offered, hours and days of operation, whether evening hours are available, and if transportation to and from the center is provided.

The third edition will be available in four volumes, broken down by region. Each volume will be approximately $70, with a discount on the purchase of all four. Obviously this is not the sort of purchase an individual would make, but your local library or chapter of the Alzheimer's Association would be likely to have a copy. You can contact Health Resources Publishing at:

Brinley Professional Plaza
P.O. Box 1442
Wall Township, NJ 07719-1442
1-800-516-4343 or 732-681-1133

Your local Office on Aging should also be a good source of information on adult day services. The Eldercare Locater at 1-800-677-1116 can give you that number; when you call, make sure to have the county and zip code of your loved one ready.

As always, your local Alzheimer's Association should be a valuable resource. Many times, members can give you the names of area centers and tell you of their experiences with them.

Financing Adult Day Center Care

As always, this is a problem area. While some counties offer grants to help defer the cost of adult day services, frequently there is a long waiting list for such assistance (as, indeed, there can be to get into the center itself). Medicare does not cover such costs. While Medicaid does not usually cover them, it may help pay for in-home medical care for the those below certain income levels, depending on the state of residence. The county social services agency, the local Office on Aging, and the Alzheimer's Association are good resources to consult regarding Medicaid benefits in the state where the patient lives.

ORIENTATION THERAPY—MAKING THE PATIENT COMFORTABLE IN A NO-LONGER-FAMILIAR SETTING

Several of the symptoms of Alzheimer's are rooted partly in the fact that the patient does not feel safe in an environment no longer seen as familiar. If you've awakened in a strange hotel room, forgetting for the moment that you're out of town, you can relate to this sense of disorientation, which brings on a variety of feelings, including fear and anxiety. Imagine feeling that way frequently during the course of a single day; this is what Alzheimer's patients experience on a daily basis. No wonder they can become frightened, suspicious of others, anxious, and agitated, and that the phenomenon known as sundowning exists, the anxiety and agitation that many patients feel as the day draws to a close.

In Chapter Seven drugs that treat these behavioral symptoms of Alzheimer's are discussed. Drug therapy should be combined with orientation therapy, with providing the patient with several clear reminders of who he is, where he is, and of the day and time. The behaviors exhibited in sundowning, for instance, can be reduced by providing cues that orient the patient to the time of day—the caregiver should refer to dinner being made and almost being ready, to other people returning home for the day, to the fact that the evening news is about to come on. These sorts of cues should be provided throughout the day. Have at least one large clock that the patient can readily see and check for the time. A large calendar helps orient the patient; what may be most helpful is something you can make yourself, a large page with just that day and date written boldly in magic marker. Having the day, date, and time prominently displayed can help cut down on that behavior mentioned very early in Chapter One of this book, the constant asking for this information that a large number of Alzheimer's patients engage in in an attempt to orient themselves and therefore feel safer.

The Memory Book—an Important Part of Orienting the Patient

The Wealshire home in suburban Chicago always has residents work with family members to prepare a large scrapbook called a memory book. This book tells the story of the resident's life, with pictures of parents, siblings, children, and grandchildren at different ages, and of important places such as the home the resident lived in as a child, the home lived in as an adult, schools attended, all clearly labeled. The patient can turn to this book and become reoriented in times of confusion and can use it at other times, such as when speaking with staff or fellow residents. A valuable tool for the resident, it is also a keepsake for the family to treasure.

A VALUABLE RESOURCE FOR PATIENT AND CAREGIVER

Elder Books of Forest Knolls, California, refers to itself as "The Alzheimer's Bookshelf," and for good reason. It offers a range of resources for families, patients, and caregiving associations. Books include stories of personal experiences, such as *Surviving Alzheimer's: A Guide for Families* by Florian Raymond, the first book written by a family caregiver, and Larry Rose's *Show Me the Way to Go Home,* a first-person narrative of a man diagnosed at fifty-four, and the inspirational *Coping with Caregiving: Daily Reflections for Alzheimer's Caregivers* by Lyn Roche.

Elder Books also features one-of-a-kind offerings that can prove invaluable to those dealing with everyday coping issues, notably activities-focussed materials. For instance, a book first published by the Alzheimer's Association of Wellington, New Zealand, has proven popular with individuals to use at home and for use in such settings as adult day centers and nursing homes; it is *Music Movement Mind and Body* by Bridget Watson, an exercise book and audio tape designed for those with dementia.

Activity books offered include *Failure-Free Activities for the Alzheimer's Patient* by Carol Sheridan, M.A., and card sets and objects designed to be used by the person with Alzheimer's. Such activity books are a godsend to caregivers trying to cope with frequently bored and restless Alzheimer's patients.

Finally, the publisher offers several books on reminiscing, a powerful healing activity for those with Alzheimer's. Reviewing their memories with the help of techniques for caregivers returns a sense of competence and value to the Alzheimer's patient. *Tell Me a Story* is a set of fifty-six cards that facilitate reminiscing and are an ideal companion to Carmel Sheridan's book, *Reminiscence.*

Orders can be placed through a toll-free number: 1-800-909-COPE.

The mailing address is:

P.O. Box 490
Forest Knolls, CA 94933
Phone: 415-488-9002
Fax: 415-488-4720
E-mail: elder@nbn.com

A RESOURCE FOR
THE HARD OF HEARING

Problems that the elderly have in understanding others and in communicating may be due partly or totally to hearing problems.

A national non-profit consumer-education group, Self Help for Hard of Hearing People, Inc., offers information about hearing aids, including the newer digital ones that, though expensive, work extremely well for some people. You may write to them at 7910 Woodmont Av-

enue, Suite 1200, Bethesda, Maryland 20814; please en-
close a self-addressed stamped envelope. The organization's web site is *www.shhh.org.* and their e-mail
address is *national@shhh.org.*

NINE

Is There a Cure in Sight?
What the Near Future Holds

WE'VE COME SO FAR SO FAST IN KNOWLEDGE—AND WE'RE GOING FURTHER

Hard as it is to believe, considering the current depth of our knowledge of dementia in general and Alzheimer's in particular, as recently as the early 1980s, those likely afflicted with Alzheimer's were getting the much more general (and therefore much less informative) diagnosis of "senile dementia."

You'll see in this chapter that the study of Alzheimer's has progressed beyond what would have been conceivable just a few years ago, due to the combining of greater public awareness with tremendous advances in medicine.

Alzheimer's has been featured as a cover story in a number of national publications, even one as popular as *People* magazine. The approach taken in that magazine has done wonders in familiarizing the public with the disease and, indeed, making it something one can speak about in public—it's the "coming out" of those whose relatives have been afflicted. Entertainers such as Mike Myers and Shelley Fabares, sports stars such as Keith Hernandez, and even the wealthy and powerful, exemplified by Jay Rockefeller—all have openly discussed the impact Alzheimer's has had on their lives. And certainly millions are aware of the situation of former President Ronald Reagan.

What's the value of awareness? Well, in addition to making all those whose lives are touched by Alzheimer's feel less isolated, it has the very practical effect of increasing research dollars spent in the quest for better treatments and a cure. The concern about Alzheimer's is underscored by the fact that the elderly are the fastest-growing segment of the population, so anything that affects them affects all of society.

This concern has taken us from a situation in which the disease wasn't even fully recognized in the 1980s to the FDA approval of not one, but two Alzheimer's-specific drugs in the past five years. And the medical aspect is not the only one showing a positive change. Why, just consider the fact that in 1987 only about six hundred adult day centers existed; ten years later, there are more than four thousand, an increase of almost 700 percent.

In this final chapter of *Is It Alzheimer's?* you'll read about the next challenge, which is also the next cause for hope—the tremendous advances that have been made in seeking a basic, molecular-level understanding of the disease. Such an understanding points not only to a possible genetic treatment, but also to the development of better traditional drugs. And yes, to underline one last time the basic point of this book: All the research done in recent years only further increases benefits of the diagnosis.

The sooner you and your family know exactly what is causing a relative's dementia, the sooner you may be able to take advantage of the treatment situation that has changed so much so recently.

First of all, while genetic testing itself is possible due only to the tremendous sophistication of our scientific knowledge, physically it's a simple procedure for the person being tested—a blood sample is taken. Yet the simplicity ends there, as various proteins in the blood sample are then isolated and analyzed. Genetic testing has been much in the news of late, due to its newness, due to the alluring possibility of cures in the relatively near future through genetic manipulation, and due to the potential for a harmful emotional and health insurance impact on those found to have defective genes. The subject is of such importance that it was the focus of the keynote address of the 1996 Annual Meeting of the New York City Chapter of the Alzheimer's Association.

In her comments, titled "Genetic Testing & Alzheimer's Disease: Ethical Issues for Providers and Families," Christine K. Cassel, M.D., directly addressed concerns of many with Alzheimer's in their family. Dr. Cassel is a Professor of Geriatrics and Adult Development at Mount Sinai Medical Center in New York, as well as Chair of that department. She also chairs the Ethics Advisory Panel of the National Alzheimer's Association.

Alzheimer's has been associated with possible abnormalities on four different chromosomes, Numbers 1, 14, 19, and 21.

The apoE gene on chromosome 19 has three alleles, or forms: apoE2, apoE3, and apoE4. Most people have the apoE3 allele and the rarest allele, apoE2, may help those who carry it live into a healthy old age. The apoE4 allele is associated with the most common type of Alzheimer's, late onset. Not everyone who carries the apoE4 allele develops Alzheimer's and that not everyone with Alzheimer's carries this allele. The genetic picture is more complicated than we are able fully to understand at this time.

Our incomplete knowledge of the role played by the apoE4 allele means that it is not yet known how to interpret the fact that someone is carrying it. Further, those who do not carry it are not assured that they will never develop Alzheimer's.

In her keynote address, Dr. Cassel made a very important point: *people relate to information in emotional ways.* For instance, you may want the information because you have an older relative with the disease, and you're curious about yourself. You're tested, and it indeed turns out that you have the form of the gene related to Alzheimer's. The next week, you misplace your check book, or the car keys, or you can't bring to mind the name of that actor whose work you've always loved.

Without having had the test, or if you'd tested negative for this allele, you'd probably brush off these events. After all, they seem to start happening to all of us in our thirties or forties, and only become more frequent as time goes by. But if you know that you have the gene, you could interpret these events in a very different way, as the beginning of an inevitable decline into Alzheimer's. How would that affect your overall outlook, and your desire to take control of your future, both medically and financially? You may despair, and throw normal caution to the wind.

There is, of course, another side to the issue. If you have been tested and found to have the gene, you may be more inspired to plan for the future, with longterm care insurance, healthcare proxies, a living will, etc. Maybe you'd even live a fuller life right now, even if you suspect that Alzheimer's is thirty or forty years off in your future.

Knowing you have the gene may, as well, enable you to take better preventive strategies. You'd probably give more serious thought to the information about prevention mentioned at the end of Chapter Seven. Further, as more is learned about medications to treat both the core disease and its symptoms, it may be discovered that certain drugs work best on those with one type of genetic makeup, while others work better on those with yet another genetic profile. A research data base of those Alzheimer's families both with and without the gene could be extremely useful in the development of protocols for new drug treatments.

As a medical ethicist, Dr. Cassel made a further, humanistic point. Genetic testing has, for instance, greatly reduced the incidence of both Tay Sachs disease and of Down's syndrome. Such reduction has not come, however, through curing the diseases, but through aborting fetuses found to have the genetic abnormalities that cause them. Tay Sachs, found in Ashkenazic Jews, causes a great deal of pain and suffering during the infancy of those who have it, as well as an early death; most people would judge it merciful not to put an infant through such pain. But Down's syndrome is different, and many of those who have either had Down's children in their own families, or grew up knowing families who did and who coped well with the condition, know the special joy such children can bring. And would one want to eliminate those who might develop Alzheimer's decades down the road? Think of the contribution of one likely sufferer alone, poet and satirist Jonathan Swift, and multiply that loss by tens of thousands.

As someone working on a daily basis in the field of genetic testing, Marvin Schwalb, Ph.D., Director of the Center for Human and Molecular Genetics at the New Jersey Medical School, has also noted areas of concern to those considering having testing. Similar to Dr. Cassel, he points out that the emotional knowledge of your genetic state can be very difficult to bear, especially since treatments for Alzheimer's work only to varying degrees, depending on the individual patient, and since there is not yet a cure in sight. In Dr. Schwalb's opinion, it would be necessary to evaluate whether the potential trauma of the information is worth a potentially positive finding, such as the fact that one is carrying the apoE2 allele that seems to protect against Alzheimer's.

Further, while some people think they can avoid potential problems with insurers by paying for such testing themselves and never telling their current insurance companies or those doctors whom they pay with insurance about potentially negative findings, Dr. Schwalb points out that this issue is more complicated than this. For instance, what if you discover that you may have a greater genetic risk of developing Alzheimer's than you had before realized. Would you lie about this information when buying insurance in the future? Aside from the ethical issue of lying itself, what if your deception is later discovered by the insurer? It is fairly certain that your coverage would be cancelled or at least altered.

Since genetic testing is going to have an even greater presence in our lives, Dr. Schwalb is certain that the day will come in the not too distant future in which state and federal legislatures will take steps to protect individuals from being discriminated against due to genetic information. That day has not quite arrived, however, and those tested now may not be covered by future legislation.

Dr. Schwalb has excellent advice for those with a first degree relative with Alzheimer's. He strongly suggests that the DNA of the relative be banked; that way, if major genetic discoveries are made that could greatly affect the disease, even if that relative has passed away, his or her genetic material would be available for the type of testing not yet available.

GENE THERAPY—THE FUTURE HOPE FOR A CURE

As more is learned about the underlying causes of Alzheimer's, there is hope for a cure, as opposed to present treatments, which basically slow the progress of the disease.

To put it in very basic terms, the current understanding of Alzheimer's is that the disease occurs due to an abnormality in the functioning of genes on one of certain chromosomes (discussed at the end of Chapter Two). Researchers think that, when a defective gene connected with Alzheimer's is activated, or "switched on," it directs the production of a substance harmful to cells in the brain. For instance, a defective gene is likely triggering the production of an excessive amount of beta amyloid, which leads to the formation of senile plaques in the brain. These plaques are a hallmark of Alzheimer's.

Optimally, gene therapy would prevent diseases from

developing in the first place; it would cure them. But treatments rather than cures are more likely at this stage, and very much sought after. In fact, the greatest promise offered by genetic research at this time is a better understanding of the biochemical steps in the disease process. This understanding could lead to more effective interventions in these steps through the use of drugs or even dietary changes.

Gene therapy involves three considerations: identifying the chromosome and then the area on the gene responsible for a problem, determining what that problem is (too much of, say, a certain enzyme being produced, or perhaps not enough), and determining how to correct it. The first two are the focus of one of today's major scientific endeavors, the Human Genome Project. The goal of this sweeping study is to map the genetic material of the body, identifying and determining the function of every area on every chromosome. The third, correcting genetic defects, calls for the introduction of altered genetic material into cells. Such a process poses a special problem with the dementing illnesses such as Alzheimer's, since the cells of the brain are involved, most likely calling for any effective therapy to cross the blood-brain barrier, a chemical "gate" that many drugs, enzymes, etc. are unable to cross. One possible way to accomplish the delivery of altered DNA into the brain is through the use of liposomes, lipid-coated sacs that may be able to cross the barrier.

Working on the genetic level is obviously a far cry from the medicine we've always known. Top notch researchers worldwide are investigating ways to make gene therapy possible. In the text *Dementia*, edited by Peter J. Whitehouse, MD, Ph.D., the following techniques that have been developed to introduce DNA into cells are discussed in Chapter Two, "The Genetics of Dementia":

1. **Transfection.** Per the text, it is the chemical process by which cells exposed to calcium will absorb small amount of DNA. Unfortunately, transfection is not efficient, resulting in only 1 in 100,000 cells integrating the DNA into its chromosomes.

2. **Microinjection.** A process involving the injection of DNA directly into the nucleus of a cell. While the process works quite well on the individual cell, it is labor-intensive and therefore limited to the treatment of only a few cells. Gene therapy, at this point in research, provides manipulation of approximately 2 percent of cells. Although this is only a small percent, gene therapy can still have an impact on a disease process; this is currently being studied.

3. **Viral-mediated gene transfer.** In this process, pieces of RNA are placed into a virus that then infects cells, where the RNA changes into DNA and alters the genes of the cell. Unfortunately, it is impossible to target specific cells using this process, a liability that could lead to malignancy in some of the cells unintentionally affected.

Despite problems with the above methods, success in introducing genetic material into the cells of live animals has been achieved in some cases; as you'll see below, at times this success can only be described as spectacular.

Some News with Special Import for Alzheimer's Sufferers

In fact, work in live animals reported on in the June 1997 issue of the journal *Nature Genetics* holds a lot of promise for those with Alzheimer's, and their families. The news involves the insertion of large pieces of human DNA into mice in laboratories in Japan. While this type of insertion has been done for several years, it has never been on this scale before—some of the mice actually have a whole human chromosome. Further, a number of the mice have been able to pass the new genetic material on to their own offspring, a groundbreaking development with tremendous implications for work with birth defects. The news that pertains to Alzheimer's patients is that the Japanese researchers are now trying to develop mice with a human chromosome 21. While they wish to do so in order specifically to study Down syndrome, you will recall that chromosome 21 has also been implicated in Alzheimer's. The work in Japan cannot help but advance our knowledge of this disease, thereby bringing us closer to more effective treatments, and a possible cure.

One Research Success Story with Promise for the Future

One possibly workable technique has come from advances in molecular biology. *The New York Times* of September 3, 1996, reported on some very promising developments. They were presented in the journal *Nature Medicine* and concerned the collaboration of researchers at Ariad Pharmaceuticals and scientists at Harvard and Stanford Universities. The scientists developed a technique to switch an abnormal gene off, insert a normal one, introduce a new switching protein that would activate the replacement gene, and then regulate that new protein's function, thereby controlling the activation of the new gene. To do so, they used drugs originally designed to suppress the immune system combined with the insertion of a package of genes into a cell.

The scientists then licensed this technique to Ariad, which used it in work on human growth hormone. In the case of a substance such as human growth hormone, abnormal genes would not have to merely be replaced with healthy ones, but the function of the replacement genes would have to be regulated, since too little of the hormone is not effective, and too much can result in gigantism. Ariad's use of the technique worked well in studies with human skin cells, first *in vitro*, and then when the cells were implanted in mice, where they continued to produce human growth hormone. Such success is only a beginning step—though an impressive one—toward using it in humans.

As with many scientific discoveries, the one leading to this approach came about while researchers were tackling another problem. In this instance, the scientists were Harvard chemist Dr. Stuart Schrieber and Stanford molecular biologist Dr. Gerald R. Crabtree, and they were investigating how certain drugs that suppressed the immune system worked. They noticed that the three immumo-suppressive drugs they were looking at all had unusual dumbbell-shaped molecules. In addition, the drugs could easily pass into cells, where they could grasp the two separate ends of an individual protein, areas referred to as *domains*, one at each end of their dumbbell shape. Perhaps, the researchers theorized, a gene could be switched off by separating its two domains, and switched back on by reuniting them, a process to be controlled by dosages of the drug. Further, as discussed above, a replacement gene could be inserted, and its activation regulated by a newly introduced switching protein controlled by the drugs. The technique resulted in Ariad's success, as previously noted.

For good reason, research in gene therapy is one of the great adventures of our age. So much is on the line—the reputations of that very competitive and proud breed, the research scientist, *and* literally billions of dollars in reward for those who succeed, as gene therapy will be to the 21st century what prescription drugs have been to our own. Our knowledge in this field is growing exponentially, and gives us every reason to look forward to the day when Alzheimer's, along with a number of other tragic diseases, is a thing of the past.

APPENDIX

Following are the two charts from the *Diagnostic and Statistical Manual of Mental Disorders, Fourth Edition (DSM-IV)* that feature the criteria doctors use in diagnosing the two most common types of dementia, dementia of the Alzheimer's type and vascular dementia.

Published by the American Psychiatric Association, the *DSM-IV* provides doctors with a complete presentation of all criteria to consider in diagnosing patients with mental disorders; it is a codification of the association's consensus regarding the factors to be assessed in order to arrive at the most reliable and valid diagnosis possible. The periodic revision of this reference is a team effort, involving the work of over a thousand individuals and of numerous professional organizations. Comprised of information based on studies and on reviews of those studies, it offers the most rigorous scientific examples of psychiatric disorders available.

The *DSM-IV* is a valuble tool for doctors who face quite a range of possibilities in the beginning of the diagnostic process when they first sit down with a patient (and in some cases, with the patient and family) and begin to take the patient's medical history. Similar to all tools, it must be used intelligently, with knowledge and flexibility. Most doctors see it as a guide to be used with clinical skill and acumen, realizing that the process of diagnosis must always, in the end, be reached by an experienced, open-minded doctor alert to the nuances of the individual patient's case.

Diagnostic criteria for Dementia of the Alzheimer's Type

A. The development of multiple cognitive deficits manifested by both
   1. memory impairment (impaired ability to learn new information or to recall previously learned information)
   2. one (or more) of the following cognitive disturbances:
      (a) aphasia (language disturbance)
      (b) apraxia (impaired ability to carry out motor activities despite intact motor function)
      (c) agnosia (failure to recognize or identify objects despite intact sensory function)
      (d) disturbance in executive functioning (i.e., planning, organizing, sequencing, abstracting)

B. The cognitive deficits A1 and A2 each cause significant impairment in social or occupational functioning and represent a significant decline from a previous level of functioning.

C. The course is characterized by gradual onset and continuing cognitive decline.

D. The cognitive deficits in Criteria A1 and A2 are not due to any of the following:
   1. other central nervous system conditions that cause progressive deficits in memory and cognition (e.g., cerebrovascular disease, Parkinson's disease, Huntington's disease, subdural hematoma, normal-pressure hydrocephalus, brain tumor)
   2. systemic conditions that are know to cause dementia (e.g., hypothyroidism, vitamin B_{12} or folic acid deficiency, niacin deficiency, hypercalcemia, neurosyphilis, HIV infection)
   3. substance-induced conditions

E. The deficits do not occur exclusively during the course of a delirium.

F. The disturbance is not better accounted for by another Axis I disorder (e.g., Major Depressive Disorder, Schizophrenia).

Diagnostic criteria for Vascular Dementia

A. The development of multiple cognitive deficits manifested by both
   1. memory impairment (impaired ability to learn new information or to recall previously learned information)
   2. one (or more) of the following cognitive disturbances:
      (a) aphasia (language disturbance)
      (b) apraxia (impaired ability to carry out motor activities despite intact motor function)

    (c) agnosia (failure to recognize or identify objects despite intact sensory function)

    (d) disturbance in executive functioning (i.e., planning, organizing, sequencing, abstracting)

B. The cognitive deficits in Criteria A1 and A2 each cause significant impairment in social or occupational functioning and represent a significant decline from a previous level of functioning.

C. Focal neurological signs and symptoms (e.g., exaggeration of deep tendon reflexes, extensor plantar response, pseudobulbar palsy, gait abnormalities, weakness of an extremity) or laboratory evidence indicative of cerebrovascular disease (e.g., multiple infarctions involving cortex and underlying white matter) that are judged to be etiologically related to the disturbance.

D. The deficits do not occur exclusively during the course of a delirium.

Reprinted with permission from the *Diagnostic and Statistical Manual of Mental Disorders*, Fourth Edition. Copyright © 1994 American Psychiatric Association.

GLOSSARY

A-beta—a recently identified component of the sheets of *beta amyloid* that make up the *amyloid* or *neuritic plaques* that are a hallmark of Alzheimer's Disease.

Acetylcholine—a *neurotransmitter,* or chemical messenger, which permits communication between neurons. It has many messenger roles, but a critical one is between nerve cells concerned with memory. Levels of acetylcholine decrease significantly in those with Alzheimer's.

Age-related cognitive decline—the mild forgetting experienced by most people as they age.

Age-related memory impairment—see age-related cognitive decline.

Allele—some genes have several forms to direct cell expression; these forms are called alleles.

Altered tau—see *tau.*

Alzheimer's Association—see Alzheimer's Disease and Related Dementias Association.

Alzheimer's disease—a progressive, degenerative disease of the central nervous system named in 1910 for the German physician who first described it as a distinct disease process. While it mainly strikes the elderly, it can also onset in middle age, and, in extremely rare cases, even earlier. It is believed to affect as many as four million Americans. As the disease process is not yet fully understood, there is no cure, but both the disease and its behavorial symptoms can be treated.

Alzheimer's Disease and Related Dementias Association (ADRDA)—the major information, support and advocacy organization for Alzheimer's disease in the United States. Its headquarters are in Chicago, but there are chapters throughout the country.

Amyloid plaques—also known as *neuritic plaques*; the dense plaques found outside *neurons*, they have *beta amyloid* at their core and are a hallmark of Alzheimer's.

Amyloid precursor protein (APP)—the lager protein from which *beta amyloid* is formed.

Antioxidants—"scavengers" of *free radicals,* highly reactive oxygen molecules which destroy cells or cause cell damage. Since antioxidants fight free radicals, it is believed that they can help slow the aging process. An antioxidant that has been shown in studies to help certain Alzheimer's patients is *vitamin E;* being an antioxidant as well, *vitamin C* may help some people with Alzheimer's. The herb ginkgo biloba, also shown in studies to help some people with Alzheimer's, vascular dementia and age-related cognitive decline has antioxidant properties.

ApoE—see *apolipoprotein.*

ApolipoproteinE (apoE)—a protein that seems to play a role in the brain; it carries cholesterol in the blood. The gene responsible for producing this protein is often referred to simply as *apoE.* Located on Chromosome 19, this gene has three *alleles*—apoE2, which is the least common, seems to protect against Alzheimer's and enable those who have it to live healthily into old age; apoE3, which is the most common; its role in Alzheimer's or protecting against it is not yet understood; and apoE4, which has been associated with a tremendous increase in the chance of developing late-onset Alzheimer's, the most common form of the disease. When produced by the apoe4 allele, apolipoprotein is implicated in the formation of *beta amyloid*, the form of amyloid found in neuritic or amyloid plaques; these plaques are a hallmark of Alzheimer's.

Aricept (donepezil)—the second drug approved by the FDA specifically to treat Alzheimer's. Like *Cognex*, it slows the breakdown of *acetylcholine* in the brain, allowing it to remain active longer than it would have otherwise.

Beta amyloid—a fragment of the larger protein called *amyloid precursor protein (APP)*, beta amyloid is found in dense deposits in the core of *amyloid* or *neuritic plaques*.

Brain cells—see *neurons*.

CAT scan—see *computerized tomography scan*.

Cerebral cortex—a thin layer of gray matter on the surface of the brain, this region is associated with such higher functions as language, reason, and judgment, though these are not the only functions it directs. Over 200 distinct areas of the cerebral cortex have been described by researchers, as well as fifty different functions. Voluntary and involuntary motor functions are controlled by this region of the brain. The cerebral cortex and the *hippocampus* are the two regions of the brain most affected by Alzheimer's.

Choline—one of the B complex vitamins, it is essential for the proper metabolism of the fats in the body and vital to the production of *acetylcholine*.

Cholinergic neurons—*neurons* that *acetylcholine*.

Cognex (tacrine)—the first drug approved by the FDA to treat Alzheimer's. It acts by slowing the breakdown of *acetylcholine* in the brain, allowing it to remain active longer than it would have otherwise.

Computerized tomography scan (CT scan or CAT scan)—a radiologic test employing a computer and x-rays to produce a detailed picture of the brain.

Confabulate—to make up events to cover memory loss. Confabulations are an unconscious defense mechanism which protects the patient from consciously acknowledging memory problems.

CT scan—see *computerized tomography scan*.

Delirium—an acute neurological disorder characterized by an abrupt onset and severe confusion.

Dementia—a neurologic disorder characterized by a slow, continuous decline from a previous level of intellectual function and by the hallmark of this impairment, which is significant memory loss. Other impairments of intellectual function include difficulty in expressing language, abnormalities in motor skills, and personality changes. The decline in these functions is serious enough to interfere with social and occupational functioning. Dementia is a symptom of an underlying disease or condition; some dementias are reversible.

Denial—an unconscious defense mechanism used to resolve emotional conflict and relieve anxiety by disavowing thoughts, feelings, or external reality factors that are consciously intolerable.

Designer drugs—drugs developed to intervene in specific steps in the biochemical process of a disease.

Ginkgo biloba—an extract from the leaf of the

ginkgo tree, found in Asia. Ginkgo biloba has been used as a medicinal herb in China for thousands of years. It has been widely prescribed in Europe in the past few decades to treat memory disorders. Ginkgo has a number of properties that make it work in some patients with memory problems. It is an *antioxidant*, so it can help fight cell damage from *free radicals*, and it reduces blood viscosity (stickiness), so it improves circulation to and in the brain, which provides vital oxygen to brain tissue.

Hippocampus—a region deep within the brain responsible for memory formation and storage; it is the first region strongly affected by Alzheimer's. The hippocampus and the *cerebral cortex* are the regions of the brain most affected by the disease.

Free radicals—the common term for *oxygen free radical molecules*. These are oxygen molecules with an unpaired electron; they readily bond with molecules in other substances, which can cause harmful chemical reactions. They have been linked to such diseases as cancer and *Alzheimer's,* and to the aging process itself. *Antioxidants* act against free radicals.

Magnetic resonance imaging (MRI)—a radiologic technique that uses magnetic fields to generate a computer image of brain anatomy.

Membrane—the outer surface of a cell.

Mitochondria—the area of a cell responsible for converting glucose and oxygen into the energy that enables the cell to function.

MRI—see *magnetic resonance imaging.*

Neuritic plaques—see *amyloid plaques.*

Nerofibrillary tangles—twisted nerve cell fibers and *paired helical filaments* found in *neurons*; they have an altered form of the protein *tau* as a main component.

Neurons—the specialized cells of the central nervous system.

Neurotransmitters—chemical messangers that permit communications between *neurons*.

Oxygen free radicals molecules—see *free radicals*.

Parkinson's Disease—a central nervous system disease of the basal ganglia which impairs coordination and may lead to dementia.

PET scan—a radiologic technique that shows the flow of glucose and oxygen through the brain; it enables researchers to see which areas of the brain are active and which are not. It reveals functions as well as structures. PET stands for *positon emission tomography*.

Positon emission tomography—see *PET scan*.

Senile dementia—a term once used to describe dementia in those over sixty-five; it is now outdated.

Single photon emission computerized tomography (SPECT scan)—a radiologic test that allows the monitoring of blood flow to different parts of the brain. It reveals both structure and function.

SPECT scan—see *single photon emission computerized tomography*.

Sundowning—the term used to describe the worsening of certain behavioral symptoms of Alzheimer's in late afternoon through the early evening, literally as the sun goes down.

Tau—a protein that, in a form called *altered tau*, is the main component of the *paired helical filaments* in *neurofibrillary tangles*.

Vascular dementia—formerly called *multi-infarct dementia* (MID), which is the most common type of vascular dementia. Vascular dementia results from impediments to blood flow to and in the brain; these diminish or entirely stop the flow of oxygen to brain tissue, damaging the *neurons* in that tissue and affecting the functions controlled by them.

Vitamin C—an *antioxidant* vitamin that can prevent damage from *free radicals;* it may help some people with Alzheimer's.

Vitamin E—an *antioxidant* vitamin shown in initial studies to be effective against Alzheimer's and vascular dementia in some people.

ROGER GRANET, M.D., F.A.P.A., has been a practicing psychiatrist for twenty years, specializing in the emotional aspects of medical illness. He is a Clinical Professor of Psychiatry at Cornell University Medical College and a Lecturer at Columbia University's College of Physicians and Surgeons. Dr. Granet is also a Consulting Psychiatrist at Memorial Sloan-Kettering Cancer Center and an Attending Physician at New York Hospital/Cornell Medical Center and Morristown Memorial Hospital, where he is Director of Consultation-Liaison Psychiatry. He has written numerous articles on psychiatry for medical journals and textbooks and has co-authored *If You Think You Have Panic Disorder* and *If You Think You Have Depression*. Dr. Granet is also a published poet with two collections of poetry: *The World's A Small Town* (1993) and *Museum of Dreams* (1998). He lives in New Jersey with his wife, Valerie, and two daughters, Courtney and Jamie, and maintains a private practice in Morristown.

EILEEN FALLON is a book publishing professional much more accustomed to the other side of the desk, with a career first as an editor at a major New York publisher, then as a literary agent. She lives in Manhattan.

Complete and Authoritative
Health Care Sourcebooks
from Avon Books

EMERGENCY CHILDCARE:
A Pediatrician's Guide   by Peter T. Greenspan M.D.
77635-9/$5.99 US/$7.99 Can   and Suzanne Le Vert

A HANDBOOK OF NATURAL
FOLK REMEDIES   by Elena Oumano Ph. D.
78448-3/$5.99 US/$7.99 Can

ESTROGEN: Answers to
All Your Questions   by Mark Stolar, M.D.
79076-9/$5.99 US/$7.99 Can

MIGRAINES: Everything You
Need to Know About Their
Cause and Cure   by Arthur Elkind, M.D.
79077-7/$5.99 US/$7.99 Can

HGH: The Promise of
Eternal Youth   by Suzanne Le Vert
78885-3/$5.99 US/$7.99 Can

HELP AND HOPE FOR
HAIR LOSS   by Gary S. Hitzig, M.D.
78710-5/$6.50 US/$8.50 Can